Celebrating Sex and Relationships Education

Sex Education Forum

Established in 1987, SEF is a unique network of 50 organisations. Conceived in an era of great negativity towards sex education, SEF has grown and developed through a time of cultural shifts and policy changes and is now the national authority on sex and relationships education (SRE).

SEF's focus has expanded from educational settings to involve other important environments, including, home, care, health, community and youth settings. SEF aims to ensure that all children and young people receive their entitlement to good quality SRE in all settings.

Main Objectives:

- to coordinate a diverse membership and provide opportunities to explore and foster a greater understanding of SRE and related topics

- to promote and raise the profile of children and young people's entitlement to SRE through policy and advocacy work

- to share information and build capacity amongst professionals to support them with planning and delivering good quality SRE

- to manage a variety of innovative projects on SRE and related topics.

Membership of the Sex Education Forum is open to organisations that:

- work on a national level

- are involved directly or indirectly in the provision or support of SRE

- are in agreement with the Forum's Terms of Reference including the Values Framework

For more information on SEF, its members, and becoming a member visit
www.ncb.org.uk/sef

Celebrating Sex and Relationships Education

Past, present and future

Proceedings of the Sex Education Forum 21st Birthday Conference

Edited by Anna Martinez

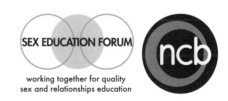

The Sex Education Forum (SEF), hosted by the NCB, is a unique network of 50 member organisations and is the national authority on sex and relationships education (SRE). We work together to ensure all children and young people receive their entitlement to quality SRE through advocacy, influencing policy and the dissemination of good practice.

NCB's vision is a society in which all children and young people are valued and their rights respected.

By advancing the well-being of all children and young people across every aspect of their lives, NCB aims to:

- reduce inequalities in childhood
- ensure children and young people have a strong voice in all matters that affect their lives
- promote positive images of children and young people
- enhance the health and well-being of all children and young people
- encourage positive and supportive family and other environments.

NCB has adopted and works within the UN Convention on the Rights of the Child.

Published by the NCB

National Children's Bureau
8 Wakley Street
London EC1V 7QE
Tel: 0207 843 6000
Website: www.ncb.org.uk
Registered charity number: 258825

NCB works in partnership with Children in Scotland (www.childreninscotland.org.uk) and Children in Wales (www.childreninwales.org.uk).

FSC
Mixed Sources
Product group from well-managed forests and other controlled sources
Cert no. SGS-COC-2953
www.fsc.org
© 1996 Forest Stewardship Council

Typeset by Saxon Graphics Limited, Derby DE21 4SZ
Manufactured in the UK

Contents

Foreword

As the newly appointed Chair of the Sex Education Forum (SEF), and what a wonderful moment in its history to take on this role, I had the task of chairing SEF's 21st Birthday Conference. I was delighted to see so many people at this celebratory event, so many old friends and supporters who have been involved with SEF's work over the last 21 years. And it really was a terrific day, with some star speakers, some wonderful presentations and practical workshops. And, despite the rumours, few us really knew exactly what the Rt Hon Jim Knight MP, Minister for Schools and Learners, was going to say when he arrived at the end of the morning session.

The day started with four plenary sessions, followed by seven workshops. Our first speaker was Anna Martinez who, as many of you will know, has been the coordinator of SEF for the last five years. She gave us a history lesson and picked out some of the highlights of what has happened in sex and relationships education (SRE) over the last 21 years. It's been quite a journey!

Our special guest speaker, Douglas Kirby, came all the way from United States to talk about the evidence that sex education actually has an impact. This is often the question that's asked: 'Yes but does it work?' His presentation helped to shake up our beliefs about what exactly is effective SRE. Listening to him, I realised that whilst much of our practice in England is very good, there is certainly room for improvement.

This was followed by an inspirational presentation from three young people, Adam Lonsdale, Alex Helliwell and Ella Durant, who were involved in the development of the Young People's SRE Charter. There was a fourth member, Esther Olayiwola, who was unable to come on the day but who made a significant contribution to the presentation, and we thank her for that. The Charter was the result of a joint initiative between SEF and the UK Youth Parliament, who co-hosted what sounded like a smashing residential. The young people's views from this consultation were also presented to the External Steering Group who conducted the review of SRE a few weeks before and made, I am told, a significant contribution to the process. Listening to their words and their passion, it is clear that the future is safe in their hands!

Finally, our keynote speaker Jim Knight MP, arrived and gave SEF the best birthday present we could ever have wanted. He announced that the government would make personal, social and health education (PSHE), which includes SRE, a statutory curriculum subject. What a historic moment – Happy Birthday SEF!

Jane Lees, Chair, Sex Education Forum

Acknowledgements

I would like to thank the following: Paul Taylor, NCB conference manager, and his team for their excellent organisation of the event; Jane Lees, for chairing the conference; and Lucy Emmerson, Lana Hashem and Fergus Crow for their support on the day. I would also like to thank all the speakers and workshop leads, including Douglas Kirby, Rt Hon Jim Knight MP, Andi Whitwham, Mark Limmer, David Kesterton, Lesley de Meza, Hansa Patel-Kanwal, Sarah Thistle, Karina Bowkett, Michelle Thompson and Chris McCabe. I would like to give a special thanks to the four young people – Adam Lonsdale, Alex Helliwell, Ella Durant and Esther Olayiwola – for their contributions and to all the young members of UK Youth Parliament for their involvement in the development of 'We Want More!', the young people's' SRE Charter for Change.

Working on the conference proceedings has afforded me the opportunity for further reflection on this historic day. I feel privileged to have worked with so many committed people. The quality of their presentations reflects the depth of their knowledge and insight into what many people consider to be a challenging subject. I am grateful that we are now able to share this learning with a wider audience.

Finally, I would like to acknowledge the hard work and dedication of all the previous coordinators and chairs, as well as SEF members, associates and civil servants. Their committment over the last 21 years has made the Sex Education Forum (SEF) into the respected and trusted authority on SRE.

Anna Martinez, Coordinator, Sex Education Forum

Overview of the day

Overall an excellent study day – What can I say? It was great to be at such an event, which will make history.

(Feedback from a conference delegate)

Celebrating Sex and Relationships Education: Past, Present and Future took place at Central Hall, Westminster, London, on Thursday 23 October 2008. This was a key moment in history, not only because it was SEF's 21st birthday but also because the first ever national review of SRE had recently concluded and the government were on the verge of responding to its recommendations.

So on the morning of the conference, amidst the media speculation and rumours, we waited in anticipation for the Minster for Schools and Learners to arrive. And it was well worth the wait. The room erupted into applause when the Rt Hon Jim Knight MP announced the government's intention to make PSHE, which includes SRE, statutory. SEF, on behalf of professionals, parents and young people, have called for statutory PSHE for many years, and it was evident by the response to the announcement that every single one of the 170 delegates in that room supported this call.

This 21st Birthday Conference, organised by NCB who host SEF, took the opportunity to look back over the changes in SRE over the years and to discuss current policy context and SEF's vision for the future.

The event was attended by professionals involved in the promotion, design and delivery of SRE, both inside and outside of school settings. Introduced by Jane Lees, Chair of SEF, the plenary sessions were opened by myself, Anna Martinez (Coordinator of SEF), and included contributions from Douglas Kirby (Senior Research Scientist and SRE expert), three young people who launched their Charter on SRE and Jim Knight MP (Minister of State for Schools and Learners). The morning offered a brief history of SRE, international evidence on effective sex education and the government's response to recommendations arising from the recent review of SRE in schools.

Seven afternoon workshops offered in-depth topical discussions in smaller interactive groups. These included: social norms and SRE; young people and pornography; building bridges between parents and school; making use of the 'Are You Getting It Right?' Pupil Audit Toolkit; Faith and Values; 'Scored project' – using football to engage young people in SRE and 17 characteristics of effective sex education. Each workshop varied in style, some focusing on a presentation based upon evidence, others more discussion-focused.

Feedback from the conference was extremely positive and many delegates felt glad to have been involved in such an important day. This publication, which is based on the presentations and transcripts from the conference, provides a report of this historic day.

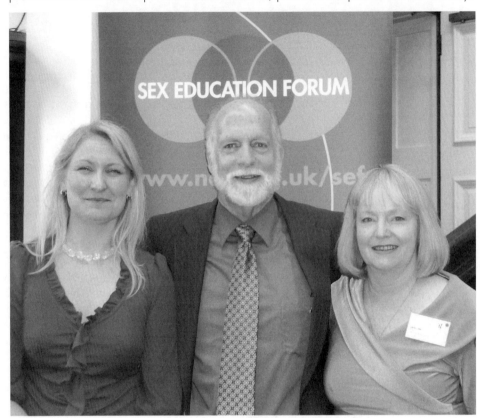

Anna Martinez, SEF Coordinator, and Jane Lees, SEF Chair, were delighted to welcome international SRE expert, Doug Kirby, to the conference.

How did we get here? 21 years of sex and relationships education

Anna Martinez
Coordinator, Sex Education Forum

1986 – 'The Moral Panic'

In 1986 there was a moral panic in the tabloid press centred on AIDS, young people's sexuality and sexual orientation. On the one hand the public were exposed to hard-hitting campaigns such as 'Don't die of ignorance' and on the other there was press outrage around some sex education materials being used in schools. One example is the Danish book *Jenny Lives with Eric and Martin* (Bosche 1983), a story about a gay couple who bring up a five-year-old girl, the daughter of Martin, that caused headlines such as 'Vile book in schools' and 'Scandal of gay porn in books read in schools' (Clyde 2001). Not unsurprisingly, this climate affected rational discussions about sex education. And in the eye of this storm, the Sex Education Forum (SEF) was conceived.

Until then young people's voices on this topic were never heard, let alone sought, and those professionals who took the view that young people needed, deserved and wanted broad-based sex education often appeared isolated. Anne Weyman, then based at the National Children's Bureau (NCB), saw the need to draw together a wide range of professionals and mobilise the broad base of support for sex education that existed. When SEF was born, in 1987, I am told that everybody in the sector let out a collective sigh of relief.

The founder eight members already reflected a diversity that continues to characterise SEF's 50 members today, and consisted of the Health Visitors Association, the Catholic Marriage Advisory Council (Marriage Care), the Health Education Authority, the National Marriage Guidance Council (RELATE), SPOD (a sexual health charity for people with disability), fpa (formerly the Family Planning Association), Brook and NCB. To hear more about SEF's birth Anne Weyman, the founder and president of SEF, will be telling her story at the birthday reception following this conference.

Now the debate on sex education was truly in the public domain. At the same time, the new Education Bill was working its way through parliament. Some Conservative peers expressed concern about the topic, claiming that homosexuality, if promoted as a valid alternative, would undermine traditional family values. As a result a new clause was introduced, requiring that, where sex education is given, 'it is given in such a manner as to encourage those students to have due regard to moral considerations and the values of family life'. The responsibility for sex education was also removed from local education authorities and given to school governors, who could now decide whether or not sex education could be taught.

At the same time that this was happening, a group of researchers met with the Health Education Authority to discuss the lack of reliable information on the sexual behaviour of the general public, information they didn't have at that time. As a result, they decided to develop the first ever National Survey on Sexual Attitudes and Lifestyles, or NATSAL. Work started on the survey, only to be stopped in 1989 by the Conservative government because of political sensitivities regarding researching sex, an area considered to be private.

1988 – Building consensus

In 1988 the Local Government Act introduced a new clause, which commonly became known as Section 28. This stated that a local authority should not promote homosexuality or promote the teaching of the acceptability of homosexuality as a pretended family relationship. Although it did not apply to schools, it served to cause confusion and anxiety amongst the teaching profession and undermined the confidence of those delivering sex education. And for those of you in the field at the time, you will know that this really did undermine people's confidence. More about that later.

Throughout the early years, SEF worked on developing a common set of values for sex education that all members could sign up to. These have, over time, evolved but still remain at the heart of all the work SEF undertakes. SEF's first publication was a simple list of resources, which proved so popular that the huge demand from professionals for support in this area could no longer be ignored. By the summer of 1990 funding was secured from the Department of Education and work with the public could really begin.

1992 – Understanding local provision of sex education

In 1992 the government launched its Health of the Nation strategy, with the reduction of teenage pregnancy and sexually transmitted infections (STIs) being two of its targets. At the same time SEF carried out a ground breaking survey of 87 local authorities; the report concluded that there existed an inconsistency in terms of the numbers of schools with sex education policies, confusion concerning the place of sex education in the National Curriculum and anxiety at all levels which had resulted in young people not receiving the sex education they needed (Thomson and Scott 1992).

1993 – Building a values framework for SRE

The 1993 Education Act included some new challenges for sex education. It stated that only the biological aspects of HIV, AIDS, STIs and human sexual behaviour could be included in the national curriculum. Parents were also given the right to withdraw their children from sex education and were not required to give a reason. The Act was followed by a long awaited circular on sex education for schools that was greeted by SEF with some optimism. It welcomed the government's commitment to the view that all pupils should be offered the opportunity to receive a comprehensive, well-planned programme of sex education during their school careers. The notion of a moral framework was also further developed in this circular.

> The Secretary of State believes that schools' programmes of sex education should therefore aim to present facts in an objective, balanced and sensitive manner, set within a clear framework of values and an awareness of the law on sexual behaviour. Pupils should accordingly be encouraged to appreciate the value of stable family life, marriage and the responsibilities of parenthood. They should also be helped to consider the importance of self-restraint, dignity, respect for themselves and others, acceptance of responsibility, sensitivity towards the needs of others, loyalty and fidelity. (DfEE 1993)

The idea of a moral framework, however, was up for interpretation.

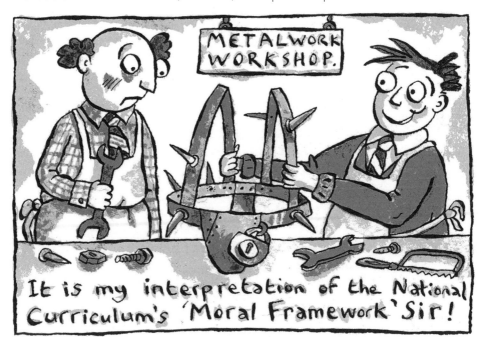

Illustration by Ant Parker.

SEF responded to this new focus by exploring values and morals from a range of perspectives, in consultation with numerous organisations including religious organisations. As a result it published its pioneering document *Religion, Ethnicity and Sex Education* (Thomson 1993).

1994 – Sex and the nation

The following year NATSAL (the first ever survey of its kind) was also published. This found that a massive 70 per cent of respondents felt that the information available to them when they first had sex was insufficient. (Johnson and others 1994)

1996 – Education Act

Two years later there was another Education Act, which consolidated all previous legislation and now expected that the biological aspects of sex education should be taught both in primary and secondary schools.

1999 – Birth of SRE

Just before the millennium, the pace really started picking up and SEF was very busy indeed. Sex education became known as 'sex and relationships education', or SRE, to acknowledge that children and young people are entitled to more than just the biological basics. The new Framework for Personal, Social and Health Education (PSHE) was published, which embedded SRE firmly within this broader programme of learning. This reflected the growing appreciation that young people do not compartmentalise their lives according to sex, drugs, alcohol and health, but rather that all of these elements are interwoven. Further, the National Healthy Schools Standard was launched, and the pioneering Teenage Pregnancy Report published, SRE being a significant element within the prevention strand. SEF was a key partner in the development of these important government initiatives, which proved to be vital levers for change.

2000 – First SRE Guidance

As a result of the growing need for clarity and support, the 2000 SRE Guidance was published. Although non-statutory, this was the most comprehensive document the government had produced on the subject and it represented an important milestone in the history of SRE; to which SEF made significant contributions. My predecessor, I am told, spent many late evenings unpicking the many responses from SEF members as part of the consultation process.

Other important events for 2000 were the equalisation of the age of consent and the launch of SEF's very first Charter for Young People (see page 108).

2001 – Just say NO to abstinence education

In 2001 we saw the launch of the national programme for the Certification of PSHE (Personal, Social and Health Education) Teaching, which was, again, a very important milestone in the history of this subject.

Also, after two study tours to the United States, SEF published its *Just Say No to Abstinence* education book (Blake and Frances, 2001), which confirmed that abstinence-only education was not a quick-fix solution to teenage pregnancy or a viable alternative to a broader, more comprehensive, programme of SRE. Later, in 2004 there was simply no appetite for programmes such as the Silver Ring Thing, who actually had to cancel events in the UK because of poor attendance.

2003 – Repeal of Section 28

After a long campaign, we saw the repeal of Section 28 in 2003, this legislation forbade the promoting of homosexuality; SEF made a significant contribution to this campaign. The Sexual Offences Act was also drafted in 2003, and aimed to clarify what constitutes a crime of a sexual nature against a child; SEF, along with other colleagues, worked hard to ensure that professionals could continue to provide information and advice without fear of criminalisation.

2006 – Beyond Biology Campaign

This year saw SEF launch its important Beyond Biology Campaign. The campaign highlighted the consensus and commitment amongst its 50 member organisations to the call for PSHE, which includes SRE, to be made a statutory subject (Martinez 2006).

2007 – UK Youth Parliament's 'Are you getting it?' campaign

In 2007 the UK Youth Parliament (UKYP) launched their 'Are you Getting It?' survey and campaign, which also called for PSHE to be made statutory.

Other significant events in this year included the launch by the National Institute for Clinical Excellence (NICE) of a two-year programme to develop PSHE guidance with a focus on sex and relationships and alcohol education, and the introduction of a revised national curriculum for secondary schools, including a new programme of study, 'Personal well-being'. Of even greater importance was the introduction of a duty on schools to promote the well-being of their pupils.

2008 – Review of SRE

So now we come to 2008 – 21 years later. The increasing groundswell of professional support for statutory SRE, the concern that SRE is not meeting the needs of over a third of young people, as well as reports from Ofsted that PSHE, although improving, was still patchy, led the government to announce a review of SRE. Once again SEF made a significant contribution to this review process, and it is with great anticipation that we wait for the Minister of Schools and Learners to tell us about the government's response to the recommendations.

So, we have seen big changes over the years, and although we know there is a lot of room for improvement, we must acknowledge all the fantastic progress that has been made in SRE. And on that note I would like to say Happy Birthday, Sex Education Forum, from all of us who have had the privilege of being involved with you over the last 21 years. I for one am very proud of your achievements, and in the words of Margaret Mead, 'Never doubt the ability of a small group of intelligent, committed citizens to change the world. Indeed it is the only thing that ever has'.

What have we learnt? What works, what doesn't and ways forward: international evidence

Douglas Kirby

Senior Research Scientist, ETR Associates

Sex education programmes have several different goals: to reduce teen pregnancy; to reduce sexually transmitted disease (STD); and to improve sexual health in the much broader scheme of things. There is far more to sexuality than simply avoiding pregnancy and STD, but what I'm going to talk about today is primarily a body of research that has focused more on pregnancy and STD prevention. I'm going to have us look back in time, and to be honest this is going to reflect my knowledge of what is happening in the United States and internationally, as well as a little bit of knowledge that I have about what has happened here in the UK.

Over 21 years ago

What did we believe and what did we subsequently learn was reality?

Belief: Knowledge equals behaviour

Twenty-one years ago what did we believe and what did we subsequently learn was reality. We believed that many teens do not have a good understanding of condoms or contraception, of STIs, HIV, pregnancy and sexual health. We believed that if we increased their knowledge they will become more likely to avoid sexual risk.

Reality

What have we found? Nearly every sex education programme that we have evaluated that measured impact upon knowledge, and there have literally been hundreds of studies that have done that, almost every one has found that these programmes do increase knowledge. Sexuality in this respect is like maths, English, history etc. – when you teach it, young people learn, of course. On the other hand, the programmes that focused primarily on knowledge did not change sexual behaviour. It turns out that knowledge is only weakly related to behaviour. That does not mean that ignorance is the answer; it isn't the answer. What knowledge does, however, is provide a foundation. Knowledge alone is not sufficient, and whilst it does provide an important foundation, there are many other factors that also need to be addressed.

15 – 21 years ago

Belief: Knowledge, values and skills equals behaviour

About 15 to 21 years ago we believed that if programmes increased knowledge and, in addition, helped clarify basic values (very basic values, not necessarily values about sexuality but values about responsibility, about care and about relationships), and if we also taught generic decision-making skills such as laying out all the possible options, thinking about the consequences of those options, maybe obtaining advice from other people, making a decision and then reviewing that decision later, and if we taught basic generic communication skills, then that combination would reduce sexual risk-taking.

Reality

Only a few studies have measured the impact of programmes that did all of the above but these didn't find any significant impact on behaviour either. As it turned out they were probably too generic and probably lacked other important characteristics needed to actually change behaviour.

Belief: Sex education should be value neutral

Another belief has been that sex education programmes should be value neutral – that they should provide accurate information and skills and then let teens decide what is best for themselves; what the right decision is for themselves. Teens themselves should decide when is the right time for them to have sex and whether or not to use condoms or contraception.

Reality

What did we find from research? That these programmes did not reduce sexual risk-taking behaviour. It turns out a very important characteristic of effective programmes is that they give a clear message about sexual behaviour. Now that does not mean that they were moralising. That does not mean that the teachers stood in front of the class and said 'Don't you have sex, it's wrong, it's sinful', etc. What it does mean, however, is that it had the young people engage in a variety of activities which allowed them to reach the conclusion that not having sex at that point in their life was a good idea. Or that if they did have sex, that they should always use condoms and contraception. And they engaged them in activities so that others in the class, peers their own age, would reinforce that message. Thus, effective programmes were not value neutral; they gave a clear message about behaviour.

Belief: Improved access to contraception leads to increased use

If programmes simply increase access to contraception, teens would be more likely to use contraception.

Reality

It is a good idea to provide access, but at least in the United States, when school-based clinics simply provided contraception, often contraceptive use did not increase in those schools. However, when the school-based clinics focused on reproductive health, as opposed to providing all kinds of primary care and giving only a small amount of attention to reproductive health, when they focused on reproductive health, when they gave a very clear message about sexual behaviour and when they did a lot of monitoring and follow-up of the young people who participated in these clinics, then contraceptive use did increase. So, simply providing access did not make a difference, but giving a clear message, focusing on reproductive health and doing a lot of follow-up did make a difference.

10 to 15 years ago

Belief: Sex education should NOT emphasise abstinence
Belief: Sex education should ONLY emphasise abstinence
Belief: Sex education that emphasises both abstinence and use of contraception will confuse young people

About 10 to 15 years ago we believed that programmes should not focus on delaying the initiation of sex because we can't stop teens from having sex. We can't stop teens; young people are going to do whatever they want to do; they're going to decide to have sex whenever they think they wish to. Some people believed that programmes should only emphasise abstinence, because if programmes talk about sex, if they provide accurate information about contraception, if they tell young people where to obtain contraception, if they teach skills to insist on using contraception, what would happen? Young people would be more likely to have sex. Some people believed that if programmes encouraged teens to be abstinent and to use contraception if they do have sex, this will only confuse them and not change any behaviour.

Reality

None of these beliefs are true. Not in the United States, other developed countries or developing countries. There's a large body of research which identified all the studies in the world meeting certain criteria. These programmes were designed for young people up to age 19 in the United States, to age 25 elsewhere, but of these almost all were 19 or under. These are curriculum-based programmes, where you have a set of pages describing the activities that should take place in the classroom as opposed to one-on-one interaction with peers, as opposed to media campaigns, or whatever. These are curriculum-based programmes with groups of youths and are focused on sexual behaviour rather than broad-based health programmes. They would be implemented in schools and could be implemented anywhere in the world. On the

9

research side, they had to have an experimental or quasi-experimental design. They had to have an intervention group and a comparison group, to collect data beforehand and collect data afterwards, to look at the change over time in the intervention group and compare it with the change over time in the control group. That way – and only that way – can we have reasonable confidence that it's the intervention that is producing the change in behaviour. They also had to have a minimum sample size, to measure impact on behaviour and had to be published in 1990 or later.

The Number of *Comprehensive* Programmes with Indicated Effects on Sexual Behaviours

	United States (N = 48)	Other Developed Countries (N = 9)	Developing Countries (N = 18)	All Countries in the World (N = 75)
Initiation of Sex				
▶ Delayed initiation	15	2	6	23
▶ Had no sig impact	17	6	8	31
▶ Hastened initiation	0	0	0	0
Frequency of Sex				
▶ Decreased frequency	6	0	2	8
▶ Had no sig impact	15	1	3	19
▶ Increased frequency	0	1	0	1
# of Sexual Partners				
▶ Decreased number	11	0	3	14
▶ Had no sig impact	12	0	5	17
▶ Increased number	1	0	0	1

Table 1

Going down the far right-hand side (see table 1), there are lots of numbers there. These are numbers of studies. So if we look in the far right-hand column we see that throughout the entire world there were 75 studies that met all of these conditions. There were 54 that measured impact on initiation of sex, and first I'm going to talk about comprehensive programmes, then I'll talk about the abstinence programmes separately.

In the United States, comprehensive programmes, means programmes that encourage young people to delay having sex, but they also encourage them to use condoms or contraception if they do have sex. We see that 23 of them delayed the initiation of sex while for 31 there was no significant impact. In regard to frequency of sex: how many times have you had sex in the last three months? We see there are 28 studies: 8 decreased the frequency; 19 had no impact; 1 increased frequency. When we look at number of sexual partners, we see that there are 32: 14 of them decreased the number of partners; 17 had no impact; and 1 appeared to increase the number of partners.

When I look at the data I reach three clear conclusions. The first is that this is very strong evidence that if you emphasise sex but also talk about condoms and contraception, this does not increase sexual behaviour. A couple of you might be looking at the 1s and saying: 'But there are two programmes there: one positive and one that had a negative impact.' The reality is, we're looking at lots of tests of significance, we're using the 0.05 level of significance. 0.05 is 5 out of a 100, 1 out of 20. Out of every 20 co-efficients 1 of them will be significant simply by chance. There are more than 60 co-efficients up there. We would expect at least 2 of them to be statistically significant in the wrong direction simply because of chance and that's what we find. So this is very strong evidence that these programmes do not increase sexual behaviour and some, but not all, actually delay the initiation of sex or reduce their frequency or reduce the number of partners. So some of them are effective, but then not all of them are.

The Number of *Comprehensive* Programmes with Indicated Effects on Sexual Behaviours

	United States (N = 48)	Other Developed Countries (N = 9)	Developing Countries (N = 18)	All Countries in the World (N = 83)
Use of Condoms				
▶ Increased use	15	1	5	21
▶ Had no sig impact	17	4	7	28
▶ Decreased use	0	0	0	0
Use of Contraception				
▶ Increased use	4	1	0	5
▶ Had no sig impact	4	1	2	7
▶ Decreased use	1	0	0	1
Sexual Risk-Taking				
▶ Reduced risk	15	0	0	15
▶ Had no sig impact	9	1	2	12
▶ Increased risk	0	0	0	0

Table 2

We turn to condom and contraceptive use (see table 2). There are 49 studies on condom use: 21 of them, or about two-fifths, actually increased condom use. We turn to contraception: of 13 studies, five of them increased contraceptive use. We turn to sexual risk-taking: 'How many times have you had sex without using a condom?' 'How many partners have you had sex with, without consistently using a condom?' These are measures that combine both sexual activity and condom or contraceptive use. Here we see that 15 out of 27, or over half, reduced sexual risk-taking.

The Number of *Abstinence* Programmes with Indicated Effects on Sexual Behaviours (US Only)

	Studies with Strong Experimental Designs (N = 6)	Studies with Weak Quasi-Experimental Designs (N = 5)	Total (N = 11)
Initiation of Sex			
▶ Delayed initiation	0	2	2
▶ Had no sig impact	6	3	9
▶ Hastened initiation	0	0	0
Frequency of Sex			
▶ Decreased frequency	0	2	2
▶ Had no sig impact	6	0	6
▶ Increase frequency	0	0	0
# of Sexual Partners			
▶ Decreased number	0	1	1
▶ Had no sig impact	6	0	6
▶ Increased number	0	0	0

Table 3

If we look at abstinence programmes, all of these studies were conducted in the United States. We need to divide them. There were those with very good research designs; that's the left-hand column. All of the studies with really strong research designs found that all six programmes failed to have any impact at all on initiation of sex, frequency of sex or number of partners. There were however five studies that were strong enough to get into this review, but their comparison groups were often a single school that was not well matched to the intervention school. So they were much weaker; it's a much weaker design than randomly assigning 20 schools and comparing one group with one other group. Of those weaker studies we see that 2 of them delayed the initiation of sex, 2 found a decrease in the frequency and 1 decreased the number of partners. So that's encouraging. Not strong evidence, but encouraging that a couple of these programmes might be effective. If we look at the impact of these programmes on condom, contraceptive use or sexual risk-taking, we see no impact at all.

Returning to comprehensive programmes, we can ask the question: 'How many of them had a significant impact on any behaviour?' And we see that 68 per cent did so. Of that 68 per cent, 5 per cent roughly is probably just due to chance. If we're going to ask, 'How many had a positive impact?', to be balanced we have to ask, 'How many had a negative impact?'. Again, 5 per cent of what we would expect by chance, so again strong evidence of positive impact. We can ask the question: 'How many had a positive impact on two or more behaviours?' There we see that about a third of them did. Those programmes, for example, delayed the initiation of sex and increased condom or contraceptive use.

So, in conclusion, regarding the impact of these programmes, what we find is that no abstinence programmes have strong evidence of positive impact; some are clearly not effective, but a couple have promising results and, in reality, there probably are a couple of programmes which do have an impact. Comprehensive programmes do not increase sexual activity, some of them delay the initiation of sex, reduce the number of partners, increase use of condoms or contraception, and some of them do all three, which I think is quite remarkable.

So that tells us emphasis upon not having sex, having fewer partners and using condoms and contraception are compatible not conflicting. It is not the case that encouraging young people to delay having sex, or not to have sex, whilst encouraging the use of condoms or contraception should they have sex is a confusing message; it's a message that young people respond to and act upon. On the other hand these programmes are not a complete solution. These programmes reduce sexual risk-taking by roughly one-third. So if in the control group 30 per cent have sex without condoms or contraception, in the intervention group that 30 per cent would be reduced to 20 per cent. So one can look at it two different ways. This glass of water is now roughly one-third full and it's also two-thirds empty; both are true, we can't deny that. So one can say, these programmes did not meet two-thirds of our need. They only worked one-third, and that is true. My view of this is that these are modest programmes. In schools they last between 5 to 10 hours; those that are effective would take between 10 and 20 hours. If a programme that modest can reduce sexual risk-taking by one-third and thereby reduce teen pregnancy and STDs by one-third, they are both incredibly effective and cost-effective programmes. On the other hand, we should not lull ourselves into believing they are the complete solution to all our problems; they're not. We still need other kinds of programmes – reproductive health services, the need to involve parents, to work with the media, to work with other groups.

Belief: Sex education programmes only work for specific groups of young people

Some people believe that programmes can only delay the initiation of sex amongst girls not boys. Programmes can only increase reported condom use amongst boys because it's the boys who really control the condoms, not the girls. Programmes can only reduce sexual risk-taking among lower risk youth because they are easier to work with or higher risk youth. Programmes are more effective with younger people before they have sex than older youth. These are common beliefs.

Reality

None of these beliefs are true. Programmes can delay sex and increase condom use among both males and females, all major racial ethnic groups in the United States, youth in both advantaged and disadvantaged communities, and both younger and older youth. I'm not saying every programme works in every case but we have multiple programmes that work for each of those groups.

Belief: Sex education can only have a short-term impact

Sex education programmes can only affect behaviour for short periods of time. It's impossible to have a long-term impact.

Reality

False. To demonstrate this I'm choosing one of the programmes that has the longest effects but this is not the only one with a long-term effect. It has ten sessions in the ninth grade (age 14–15) , ten sessions in the tenth grade (15–16) and ongoing school-wide components that may reinforce those messages in the eleventh (16–17) and twelfth (17–18) grade. And it had an impact on sexual risk behaviours for 31 months, almost three years. It actually may have had an impact for longer than that, but we stopped following the young people at that point in time.

Belief: We don't really know what constitutes effective sex education

We don't really know what constitutes effective sex education.

Reality

Yes, we do. We literally took those programmes that had very strong evidence of impact and we obtained their curricula and put them in a pile. We took those programmes that had very strong evidence that they did not change behaviour, obtained some of their curricula and put them in a pile also. Then we very carefully analysed them. What we found was that there are 17 characteristics (see page 76), which distinguish those programmes that effectively change behaviour from those that do not. These are standing the test of time. As research keeps coming out, I keep going back and looking at these 17 characteristics and the results and new research tend to support them. They are supported by research not only in the United States but internationally as well. They are also consistent with summaries of research on smoking, substance use and other fields.

Now, there is also a belief that if we implement a programme that has been demonstrated to be effective in another part of the country, it won't be effective in MY community, with MY youth. Somehow a lot of us feel that our communities are different, our schools are different, our youth are different than the youth that have been evaluated in studies.

Reality

Programmes are often effective if they are implemented with somewhat similar populations of youth and with fidelity. There are multiple studies of the same curriculum implemented and evaluated by different research teams in multiple places, which consistently find that the programmes remain effective if they are implemented with fidelity. If you cut out half the activities, then no impact. If you cut out all the condom activities, no impact on condom use. If you implement them with fidelity, all the activities as planned, they have an impact in multiple areas.

Belief: You cannot influence young people's behaviour

There are too many factors affecting teen sexual behaviour that we cannot control, for example media, and we cannot dramatically reduce teen pregnancy, childbearing or sexually transmitted infections.

Reality

We know that school-based comprehensive programmes CAN contribute to the reduction of unprotected sex, which may lead to unintended pregnancy, STDs and HIV. However, and as I mentioned before, effective initiatives should also involve families, reproductive health services and the media.

Conclusion

We've come a long way in 21 years, and in this period of time we've learned a huge amount. We've learned how to have an impact on behaviour and my conclusion then is let's put what we've learned into practice.

What do we want to see in the future? The launch of the Young People's Charter for SRE

Adam Lonsdale, member of Youth Parliament for East Riding of Yorkshire

Alex Helliwell, youth representative, UNICEF
Ella Durant, member of Youth Parliament for South Somerset

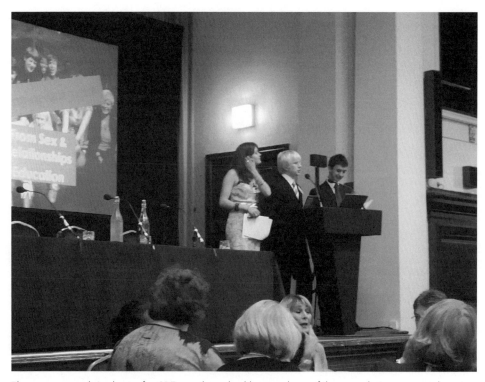

The young people's charter for SRE was launched by members of the consulation group who were involved in its development.

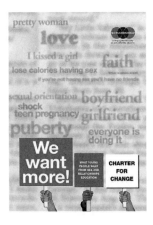

This charter is reproduced in full on pages 109–116.

The consultation

ADAM LONSDALE: We are here today to launch the new Young People's Charter. In August 2008, 15 young people went down to Brockenhurst for a two-day residential where we did activities to find out:

- where young people learn about sex
- what makes good and bad SRE
- how it can be improved
- why we need SRE
- how SRE can contribute to the five Every Child Matters outcomes
- recommendations on what schools can do

Where do young people learn about sex?

Media

Young people get messages about themselves from a variety of sources, each having their own biased view, but media is the biggest influence on young people. Through magazines, television, radio, internet and newspapers, the media tends to operate under a 'sex sells' policy. You can see this in magazines: for example, girls' magazines focus on sex as being part of love and a good relationship, whereas when you look at guys' magazines they see girls are just like sex objects that you should use.

Pornography creates false images. Also, athletes use their bodies in adverts. And, finally, magazines with problem pages can also create more false images about sex and relationships.

Society and culture

Looking at society and culture, there are plenty of mixed messages about sex, relationships and teenage pregnancy. Parents for example have a lot of misconceptions, such as 'AIDS kills', and also around contraception. There's also peer pressure, like losing your virginity before you're 16. There are gender expectations and unwritten rules about what you have to be to be a man or what you have to be to be a woman, and those are from birth. You can see them: boys are dressed in blue, girls are dressed in pink. They're misleading stereotypes that are not true, such as women with revealing clothing are obviously promiscuous and any camp man is obviously gay.

We learn about relationships, sex, sexuality and gender from a variety of sources but we want information we can trust.

Our rights

The right to SRE is contained within the UN Convention on the Rights of the Child.

ALEX HELLIWELL: For Britain and the British government to abide by the UN Convention on the Rights of a Child, they need to provide SRE. This convention is applicable to anyone under the age of 18 and was ratified by the UK in 1991.

Good health for all

State Parties shall

…ensure to the maximum extent possible the **survival and development of the child**. (Article 6.2)

…recognize the right of the child to the enjoyment of the **highest attainable standard of health** and to facilities for the treatment of illness and rehabilitation of health … strive to ensure that no child is deprived of his or her right of access to such health care services (Article 24).

…to develop preventive health care … **family planning education and services**. (Article 24).

So, being healthy, the third point there. It's probably the quintessential thing for why the UN see SRE is here to make sure people are healthy and have the highest standard of health. And they specifically mention this in Article 24, family planning education.

Why do we need SRE to be healthy? It's because sex is a risky business and relationships are a risky business. So to stay healthy we need to avoid STIs, HIV and pregnancy. We're also talking about relationships, about how to avoid a violent or an abusive relationship, issues which we think are very important.

Education for all

> State Parties shall
>
> ...**recognize the right of the child to education**, and with a view to achieving this right progressively and on the basis of equal opportunity. (Article 28)
>
> ...**without discrimination of any kind**, irrespective of the child's or his or her parent's or legal guardian's race, colour, sex, language, religion, political or other opinion, national, ethnic or social origin, property, disability, birth or other status. (Article 2)
>
> ... **recognize that a mentally or physically disabled child should enjoy a full and decent life** ... ensure that the disabled child has effective access to and receives education, training, health care services, ... conducive to the child's achieving the fullest possible social integration and individual development.... (Article 23)

Everyone deserves an education regardless of who they are. You have a long list in the second point, but one thing we felt was that disability sometimes poses an obstacle, like we heard the story of a mother denying her disabled son SRE because she didn't feel that he would live long enough to have sex. So we need to make sure it is for everyone. And applicable for all people, especially those who may need different types of help, such as those who aren't heterosexual.

Information and views

> State Parties shall
>
> ...ensure that the child has access to information and material from **a diversity of national and international sources, especially those aimed at the promotion of his or her social, spiritual and moral well-being and physical and mental health**. (Article 17)
>
> ...shall assure to the child who is capable of **forming his or her own views the right to express those views** freely in all matters affecting the child, the views of the child being given due weight in accordance with the age and maturity of the child. (Article 12)

We have the right to get information that will help us. That information needs to be reliable, and as Adam said earlier, the media has very negative images and sex sells and that doesn't give us a very reliable source of information.

We need our views and opinions heard. We are old enough to form an opinion therefore we should be heard. We know what we want and what we need, so you need to provide that for us.

What young people need

To achieve well-being and the five Every Child Matters outcomes, we need SRE

ELLA DURANT: We've created this Charter through a variety of groups across England, so it's diverse and inclusive and I will be highlighting the key points. The way SRE is taught is important and we need to improve the way it's taught, especially on the relationship front. The Charter is my hope to do this. The new Charter varies from any in the past because it incorporates the five Every Child Matters outcomes, so it makes it more relevant.

To enjoy and achieve, we need to learn about...

Relationships. SRE should be compulsory for young people. Some people don't want their children to have SRE but they should, especially the relationship side of it. If people learn about all types of relationships, we can cut down on homophobia and discrimination. We need to learn about disabled relationships, lesbian, gay, bisexual and transgender (LGBT) relationships, about people who choose to abstain and the beliefs of different religions. Young people get bullied due to misunderstanding of relationships and different types of sexual decisions. Young people need to know how to handle a relationship. Some people don't know what a successful relationship should entail and a lot of young people have friendship fallouts. If they could get proper relationship education, this could be avoided.

Young people aged five should be taught about relationships. They should be taught about what a successful relationship entails, therefore when they get older there will be less chance of homophobia and other types of discrimination and bullying.

To stay safe, we need to learn about...

How to be safe. Once you've crossed the line in a relationship, sometimes it's hard to turn back. Young people need assertiveness skills for all counts of life, not just in this, so it would be really useful if this was taught in SRE. Also, you need to know that contraception is not 100 per cent effective and maybe it's best to use different methods. Some people don't really understand about contraception. And people need to realise that girls and boys should both bear equal responsibility for contraception and that you're not a prostitute or a slut or whatever if you carry condoms with you. And we need to cut down on underage sex. With effective SRE, which is outlined in this Charter, this should hopefully happen.

We need to cut down on homophobia. Some people don't have a proper understanding of homophobia or relationships. Some young people might have two mums or two dads, this is normal for them, but some people don't really understand this and they need to be taught this.

To be healthy, we need to learn about...

STI's. You need to know how to recognise STIs and how you actually catch them. That you don't just sit on a toilet seat and get an STI. And you need to know how to tell if you're ready for sex. Some young people don't have the confidence to know what's right for them. They need to be taught this in SRE and know that *not* everybody is doing it.

And you need to know that information is confidential. You can go to a clinic and they are not allowed to tell anybody else that you've been there.

To achieve economic well-being, we need to learn about...

The costs of having a baby. You need to understand the full responsibility of actually having a child and you need to know that if you do have a baby when you are at a young age, or at any age, how to make sure that you and your child don't end up in poverty. You need to have this taught properly in SRE. And have directories handed out so people know where they can go to get help.

To make a positive contribution, we need to learn about...

Helping others. To make a positive contribution, you need to understand how other people might feel, if you say certain things to them. You need a proper understanding of relationships. You need to know how to help your friends if your friends approach you when they can't approach somebody else. And who to go to if you then need help, to help your friends.

We should have specialist, trained people in schools to deliver SRE. Some schools don't have the proper resources so we need to make sure that schools are all delivering the same level of SRE. SRE is for young people, so it should be relevant to what they need. Confidential questionnaires for feedback could be useful.

Our vision for the future

We want to see all young people get their right to SRE, so we recommend ... the earlier SRE starts the better

ALEX HELLIWELL: What is our vision for the future? For people to stop saying that their SRE was too little too late. So it shouldn't matter whom the child is, where they've come from, where they're going, they all need this education. As we heard earlier, we live in an increasingly sexualised world and without this education, they're not sure what to do.

So what do we mean by too late? Primary school. Children need to be taught in primary school – and before any of the people in the media go out and write we're suggesting teaching gay sex at five, which was a media headline in one newspaper –

we want to focus on relationships. What is good in a relationship, what is bad in a relationship. We are not just talking about intimate relationships, but also relationships with others, with parents, with peers, with teachers. So the younger the better, so children start learning about it and then will accept different kinds of relationships.

Let's talk about sex

ELLA DURANT: Let's talk about sex. Good SRE should be inclusive of all types of relationships.

The classroom environment should be safe. You should feel comfortable to talk and be able to ask questions effectively. Teachers should allow pupils to contribute. Some people have their own experiences, which could be beneficial to other young people in their classes.

We need *more* lessons and more resources and more variety. We need both practical and theoretical, not just being talked at and watching videos. That's not going to make you pay attention. It just makes you sit down and go to sleep and not really care what you're being taught. Maybe have condom demonstrations, opportunities to try it out yourself so you know how to do it effectively and then you might have less splits and cut down on teenage pregnancy later on down the line.

Pupils should be aware of resources they can get outside school, if they want to learn more, on where to go and who to get them from.

Training, timetabling, teaching

ADAM LONSDALE: SRE is just as important, if not *more* important, than the other subjects like maths and science and should be treated so and given enough time.

Students can tell when a teacher wants to be there. It is like some kind of sixth sense we have and it only makes sense that if students want to learn, they should have teachers that want to teach.

Teachers should be trained, because training makes the difference between good and bad SRE.

We need better SRE NOW!

We live in a changing and changed world. The views and ideals held ten years ago hold no water today and it's imperative that the deliverers of SRE realise this. It is also important that children are taught about relationships other than heterosexual ones. So that the stigma surrounding sexual orientation will be eradicated; so that this generation of young people will grow up understanding that everyone is equal, no matter what their sexuality.

The SRE taught in schools may be the only reliable information some pupils will receive. This can be because parents might have misconceptions or that they might just be too embarrassed to talk about it. Therefore, it is of the utmost importance that a wide range of topics are covered within SRE. We all experience relationships and sex at some time in our lives, so the better prepared we are, the better choices we make, and the earlier you learn, the more you remember.

Finally, listen to young people – we know what we need!

What is the future for SRE? The government's response to the Review of SRE in schools

Rt Hon Jim Knight MP
Minister for Schools and Learners

It's a real pleasure and an honour to follow those inspirational young people. The work that we've been doing on SRE, and the review that we've just completed and are publishing a report on today was really instigated by the work that young people did, principally through the Youth Parliament, the UKYP. Hopefully through our response they can hear that in some part at least we are listening.

And I'm also delighted to wish SEF a very happy 21st birthday. I'm particularly grateful to Anna Martinez for the work that she did in our group carrying out the SRE Review. She was extremely helpful as an expert for us in carrying out that work.

It's customary and almost tempting to start speeches with humour and gags. Probably especially following my appearance on Channel 4's *Sex Education Show* – for those who saw it! But sex education is an extremely important and serious subject, so I'm going to resist that temptation. It's a subject we shouldn't shy away from. It's a crucial part of growing up. Our approach to relationships, the choices we make and our ability to keep ourselves safe, is what marks us out as independent, free-thinking adults.

Youth is a unique time – one to be enjoyed!

An eminent Victorian author might have described growing up as 'the best of times and the worst of times'. In 1945, the *New York Times Magazine* published a solution. A teenage Bill of Rights, which they described as a ten-point Charter, framed to meet the problems of youth, rather like a teenager's Ten Commandments. It's not all that different from what we aspire to for young people today. For example, the right to have a say about their own life. Some aspects of language might have changed: the right to a fair chance and opportunity and the right to professional help whenever necessary. Some are a bit less explicit in what they say, but no less important: the right to make mistakes and find out for oneself; the right to be at the romantic age; the right to struggle towards one's own philosophy of life. But they all seem to strike an excellent balance, acknowledging that teenagers are young adults, that youth is a unique time and to be enjoyed. And that young people are still growing and developing, struggling towards their own philosophy of life.

It also underlines the fact that there's something universal about the condition of the teenager as perpetuated throughout history. The second birth of adolescence that Rousseau described when writing in the eighteenth century, with its change in temper, frequent outbursts of anger and perpetual stirring of the mind, of course given very modern visual form in Harry Enfield's Kevin of the nineties, Vicky Pollard of *Little Britain* and, obviously, the wonderful Catherine Tate, who's decidedly not bothered, or 'bovered' I should say.

But the history is not just in the hormones and it's not just about teenagers. It's also about children. The teenage Bill of Rights was published in the same week that Anne Frank was incarcerated. Young people over 50 years ago were dealing with very different things to young people in 2008. And for all that they had to endure, they have been described as 'youth without youth'. But for all the differences over the last half-century, we are seeing the same description of young people today. Mass marketing aimed at children. Celebrity and image-conscious culture. T-shirts for girls as young as six reading: 'So many boys. So little time'. Youth without youth, albeit for very different reasons. We could do worse than to look again at the ten point Charter of 1945 and its reminder of the right to learning, the right to question the values and trends of the society you're living in and – most of all – the right to have fun and all the experiences that youth should bring, but safely.

Sex … we're not all that good at talking about it

The problem is, for all the sex in our society, we're not all that good at talking about it. Parents, teachers, ministers, even on the *Sex Education Show*, there's a cultural divide when it comes to young people themselves. Around the time that the teen Bill of Rights was published, more public forums for discussing sex were starting to develop, such as *Seventeen* magazine, established in 1944. Since then girls have created whole institutions which help them talk about sex: magazines, agony aunts, sleepovers. For boys, it's not really part of the culture. Although a number of lifestyle magazines have come onto the market for men in recent years; *GQ*, *FHM* and so on, they tend to be aimed at somewhat older boys rather than teens, and I don't think are entirely intended for educational purposes. And, you don't tend to find boys talking much to each other about matters of the heart. According to popular psychology; men don't even like to ask directions, let alone for advice about sex. As a 15-year-old boy, all you've really got is the top shelf, half truths and rumours from your mates and making it up as you go along. You might call it a more vocational learning route.

But leaving it to experience is too late. In the classic comedy series *Blackadder Goes Forth*, one of my absolute favourites, Blackadder declares himself to be: 'a fully rounded human being with a degree from the university of life, a diploma from the school of hard knocks and three gold stars from the kindergarten of getting the shit kicked out of me'.

Our education system must prepare young people for life

Our children's social and emotional development should not be as haphazard as that. By the time they get to the university of life, it's too late. Our education system must prepare young people for life as fully rounded human beings and not shy away from that task. That is, after all, what education is for. To develop our critical faculties. To help us make the right choices, not just in our studies but in life. Because it's those critical faculties and the ability to make the right decisions independently that we will rely on in adulthood to keep us healthy, successful and safe. That's particularly important as young people are experimenting with other things – with alcohol, drugs, cigarettes – and operating within different social situations and the parameters of peer pressure. The right information helps us make the right choices, and that information has to come before they find themselves in the situations, with enough time to think about how to respond.

As we've seen during this financial crisis, the average person tends to make the worst decisions when they don't have the right information, when they're under pressure and when they're not able to assess the long-term implications of a decision.

Those conditions make people act irrationally and make bad choices. Although our teenage pregnancy rates are falling, they're still high compared to other countries, and 35 per cent of sexually active teens have had sex after drinking too much. That's a bad choice. One that could be avoided by warning young people of the dangers of alcohol, as well as talking to them about safe sex. Most importantly, education counters myth. It's really worrying that some young people are starting to have sex believing that you can reuse a condom if you can wash it, that you can't get pregnant during a first time, or that you're okay if you're standing up. If they were left to discover the truth at the school of hard knocks, teenage pregnancy rates would rocket.

Making PSHE statutory

This is why we've decided, following the SRE Review, that I co-chaired with real strong support, and I'm very grateful to Joss McTaggart from the UKYP and Jackie Fisher from Newcastle College, to make PSHE statutory.

At the moment, reproduction and STIs are taught as part of biology lessons and the personal and social side, as you know, as things in the non-statutory PSHE. But by making PSHE compulsory, we can make sure that young people are getting consistent teaching in sex education. We can make sure that they get more than just a biology lesson, but real lessons in life; dealing with certain situations, emotions and decisions, exploring the complex issue of sexuality and the different types of relationships in the 21st century. Struggling towards a philosophy of life.

We've got to get better at talking about sex

Making PSHE compulsory is a concrete and vital way of helping schools to meet the new duty to promote pupils' well-being. But if we're really going to make sex education better, of course it's not enough just to make it statutory. We've got to get better at talking about it. We need to support teachers. So we've asked TDA, the Training and Development Agency for Schools, to look at how we might provide better training for teachers at all stages: initial teacher training, inset and continuing professional development, and we're looking at developing a specialist PSHE role for teachers. We're also going to produce updated guidance on SRE to help teachers prepare material and we'll encourage them to use specialist professionals from outside so that pupils get a better quality education in those issues.

But it's not just teachers who need a bit more support. All of us need a bit of help to talk about sex with our own children, to get it on the agenda in our local communities, and to make sure it's approached confidently and sensibly by young people themselves. Most importantly, we want SRE to help build a real partnership between parents and their children as they approach these issues.

At the moment, almost a third of teens say that sex is not discussed openly at home. We want to help parents address these issues with their children. I know that some people worry that talking about sex will perhaps give young people ideas and they will suddenly run off and do it. But the fact is that they're having those ideas anyway. It's also a fact that children whose parents talk to them honestly about sex and relationships are less likely to have sex before 16 and more likely to use contraception when they do.

Talking about joining the army doesn't mean you're going to sign up, but when they do you wouldn't send them into battle without body armour and a bit of briefing. Surely it's better for our young people to get their briefing from us. From parents and professionals, rather than the hushed rumours of the locker room or avid chat on instant messenger. Surely it's better to rely on facts in the classroom rather than myths in the playground. Those conversations early on will pave the way for greater trust, openness and honesty in the future, where children can ask questions and parents can answer confidently without being embarrassed.

Adults should prepare children for the future

So, for Rousseau's second birth of adolescence we need a bit of a rebirth for social and emotional education. That means good sex education for every young person, not just those whose schools are good at delivering it. To go back to the teenage Bill of Rights, there's just one point out of the ten that I would disagree with. That is the right to let childhood be forgotten. In the children's plan, we committed to making this country the best place in the world for children and young people to grow up in and if we succeed, childhood will be enjoyed and not hastily forgotten in a series of bad experiences or a rush to grow up.

Childhood and adolescence will be reserved as a period in their own right – to enjoy, to celebrate, and to prepare young people for the future.

In 1883 a military writer wrote that the strength of a nation lies in its youth. He was talking about the strength of its armies, but today the point applies to our moral and intellectual strength. The younger generation are the future. The older generation need to help them to prepare for it. Not just by teaching them the skills to enable them to do a job, but by equipping them for life, and enriching their experiences.

Questions for the Minister

JANE LEES: Thank you very much for that. I'm almost lost for words. You certainly don't need help in talking about sex. We've seen the proof. And you've given us all – children, young people, teachers, sexual health workers, everybody here, including SEF – the best present we could have. So thank you very much.

JIM KNIGHT: I did want to save it up for today as a birthday present. Maybe it worked.

QUESTION: Making PSHE statutory, which obviously would include SRE, is a fantastic decision. Can you just give us a bit of a timetable as to when this might occur?

JIM KNIGHT: Sadly it's not something we can do overnight. There's some things that we can try and get overnight. And I think the signal this sends to headteachers, for example, about the importance that we place on PSHE, is something that we can try and build on very, very quickly. But in terms of the statutory curriculum being taught, I'm afraid we're probably looking at 2010. There's a period that we've got to go through. We've asked Sir Alisdair Macdonald, who is the headteacher at Morpeth School in Tower Hamlets, a fantastic school, to do a little bit more work beyond what the review did in helping us to reach this historic moment of agreeing a principle of statutory PSHE. We want him to just lead a little bit more work in how we implement that in a way that's sensitive to the various school environments that we've got and the various ages and how we properly make that home/school relationship work so that parents feel comfortable and involved in the decisions about what is taught when.

We will then have to consult on a programme of study, and get that agreed and then implemented. As you know, with anything to do with changing the curriculum, it's a bit like turning around that proverbial tanker, so it takes a frustrating period of time. I think 2010 is as quickly as we can do it.

QUESTION: What do you think we can do as practitioners? What do you think we can do as … from the Drug Education Forum, with SEF, with the PSHE Association, along with you, to capture the hearts and minds of the public to support the announcement that you've just made?

JIM KNIGHT: Well I think things have started to shift actually. I mean, we saw with some of the reporting this week and the work that Channel 4 did with the *Sex Education Show*, that we're … and there was a survey the BBC did today … we're seeing from parents a real appetite to improve things. That is something that we can build on. I think whilst undoubtedly and inevitably there may be some parts of the media that will just want to report that we've strangely announced that we're going to teach sex to five-year-olds. We try to be clear that this is going to be age-appropriate in terms of how it's implemented, and that people here aren't going to want to teach five-year-olds the detailed mechanics of sex, but people will try and run that sort of headline. Some newspapers will, but most won't I think. Most understand that there's an important issue that we're trying to address here. But if you can be working through your various networks and your associations, I think principally with parents and just having them understand what best practice looks like that exists at the moment. Because in the end that's what we're trying to do. We're trying to get best practice to be common practice.

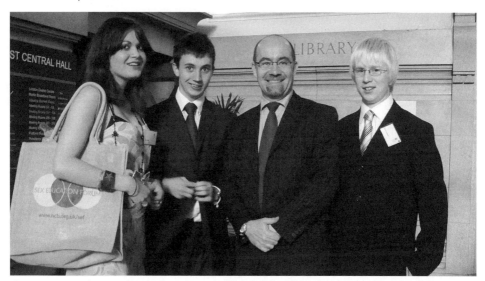

The young speakers at the conference were delighted to hear Jim Knight announce that SRE, as part of PSHE, would become part of the statutory curriculum

Workshop 1: Social norms and SRE – sharing examples from schools in Bedfordshire of the normative approach

Andi Whitwham, Drug, Alcohol and Sex and Relationships consultant, Bedfordshire

Andi.Whitwham@rhouse.co.uk

The aim of the workshop was to explore the social norms approach to SRE using a case study of schools in Bedfordshire. Participants also had the opportunity to think about what makes effective social norms messages and the challenges schools can face when adopting this approach.

What are social norms?

Social norms are a set of behavioural models and rules that are assimilated within a society.

Social norms consist of rules of conduct and models of behaviour prescribed by society. They are rooted in customs, traditions and value systems that gradually develop in this society.

Social norms affect individual activities as a whole: our personal, family and working lives. They are often of regional or national nature and display great diversity on a geographical level (dress, taboos, eating habits, the role of the family).

The social norms approach

Normative approaches help children and young people understand what their peers are doing, and these are generally positive behaviours. This approach has been developed to counteract findings that show that people of all ages generally think there are fewer healthy and more risk-taking behaviours than is actually the case (de Silva and Blake, 2006).

Why use a social norms approach?

- Perceptions held are often misperceptions
- The healthy majority think they are in the minority
- The unhealthy minority think they are in the majority
- Young people tend to underestimate the healthy choices and overestimate risk behaviours
- Normative or social norms approaches within PSHE promote positive behaviours

(Perkins, 2003)

Social norms approaches: What do they do?

Social norms approaches use a range of localised data sources to identify the social norms amongst a population and to promote a positive message about children and young people's behaviour (de Silva and Blake, 2006).

- They offer legitimacy to choices which some would feel unacceptable
- They reduce the power of longstanding myths
- They promote publicly accepted norms
- They promote trust amongst adults, children and young people
- They build on the tendency to want to be 'part of the crowd'

A step-by-step guide to a social norms approach

- Assess prevailing norms. What do children and young people believe about behaviours?
- Select the normative messages. What do children and young people want to know and what is the message for them?
- Test the normative message with the target group
- Select a delivery 'strategy'
- Undertake the message delivery
- Evaluate its effectiveness

Effectiveness of the approach

- Messages need to focus on a majority behaviour or belief (more than 50 per cent)
- Only one message subject should be chosen, allowing maximum impact
- Narrowing the frame for the campaign or intervention will help focus the message
- Understanding and working within the local context is critical to success
- Work in partnerships with young people across health, education and voluntary sectors to answer the question: 'What are the norms on different behaviours?'

Bedfordshire pilot scheme

Case study: School A

The school is a culturally diverse community, with about half of the students coming from a wide variety of ethnic backgrounds and almost a third learning English as an additional language. Significant social and economic deprivation factors affect the whole community. Eligibility for free school meals is well above the national average. A high number of students have learning difficulties and disabilities.

The school is situated in a 'hot spot' area for high teenage pregnancy, crime and drug and alcohol use.

PSHE delivery

The coordinator of PSHE is an excellent practitioner, having completed the national programme for CPD in PSHE two years previously. She recently moved to the school as Schools Sports Coordinator (SSCO) and PSHE coordinator. The school also decided to deliver PSHE through the humanities department of which she was part.

SRE delivery

A completely new PSHE programme was developed for Years 9 and 10 using activities developed by the SRE consultant and the coordinator. The SRE programme included seven lessons, ranging from STIs, contraception and relationships. The use of an excellent and highly respected school nurse, a session delivered by a pregnancy crisis and abortion centre and two theatre performances from two companies, supported the programme. The first theatre performance for Year 9 covered a range of topics including STIs, relationships, contraception and sexuality whilst the second, for Year 10, focused on dealing with teenage pregnancy. Both performances included workshops where young people could ask questions of the characters in the form of hot-seating.

The Social Norms survey was first completed in October 2007 by Year 9, 10 and 11 students. The coordinator considered herself to be the best person to work with the students in completing the questionnaire as she was highly respected and felt they were more likely to be 'honest with her' than with some of their tutors!

The second questionnaire was completed at the end of the summer term 2008 upon completion of the full SRE programme.

Case study: School B

The students are drawn from a wide catchment area within a large town in the south of the county. The majority of students are from relatively middle class, white backgrounds with low eligibility for free school meals compared to other schools. Around 14 per cent of students have learning difficulties and disabilities, which is slightly below the national average. Approximately 7 per cent are from minority ethnic groups and about 2 per cent do not have English as their first language.

PSHE delivery

The coordinator of PSHE is an excellent practitioner who believes strongly in the importance of the subject. The challenge lies with the fact that large numbers of tutors do not see it as their role to deliver PSHE and in particular SRE and drug education. PSHE is currently delivered by all form tutors, although there is a strong move for the specialist delivery of SRE and drug education by more enthusiastic members of the RE/Citizenship team next year (2009).

SRE programme

The coordinator has worked extremely closely with the SRE consultant for the past three years on training peer educators from Years 12 and 13 to deliver the majority of lessons in tutor time. The lessons they delivered to support the SRE programme covered, specifically, condom demonstrations, STIs, contraception, relationship work and access to support agencies. Year 9 received a Theatre in Education performance covering issues around condom use, relationships, sexuality and sexually transmitted infections whilst Year 9 tutors delivered pre and post follow-up work to support the performance. Peer educators delivered the vast majority of the SRE lessons in Year 10.

The Social Norms survey was first completed in October 2007 by Year 9, 10 and 11 students. Peer educators were briefed on how to support all students in completing the questionnaire, with tutors supervising the classroom environment only. Messages were devised and displayed on the school message board system.

The second questionnaire was completed at the end of the summer term 2008 upon completion of the SRE programme.

Case study: School C

The school handles 13-18 year olds and is a specialist arts college of larger than average size. A large majority of the students are white British and the proportion eligible for free school meals is below the national average. The level of student attainment upon entry to the school is broadly average. The percentage of students with learning difficulties and/or disabilities is just below the national average and the proportion of statements of special educational needs is well below.

PSHE delivery

The coordinator of PSHE is an excellent practitioner who believes strongly in the importance of the subject. The challenge lies in being responsible for at least three other key subjects or initiatives in the school. Additionally tutor delivery time for PSHE has been reduced to two, half-hour sessions. Extra time is given to Peer Education and specialist delivery of theatre in education or presentations by agencies. PSHE is currently delivered by all form tutors, but delivery can be deemed patchy in places. The school currently does not have access to a school nurse.

SRE education programme

The coordinator has worked extremely closely with the SRE consultant for the past five years on developing the PSHE and, specifically, training peer educators from Years 12 and 13 to deliver SRE, including work on contraception, STIs and relationships. The lessons they delivered to support the SRE programme covered condom demonstrations, STIs, relationship work and access to support services. The Year 10 programme was supplemented by a Theatre in Education production on teenage pregnancy.

The Social Norms survey was first completed in October 2007 by Year 9 and 10 students. Peer educators delivered the majority of the SRE lessons. Messages were devised by peer educators and displayed on the schools intranet system. All students could access these messages as individuals logged onto the computer system.

The second questionnaire was completed at the end of the summer term 2008 on completion of the SRE programme.

Introductory research for this project

December 2006–August 2008

- Initial contact by email with Wes Perkins from 'Peas in the Pod' conference in December 2006
- Adaptation of social norms questionnaire and development of SRE questions
- Adaptation of guidance manual for teachers
- Five upper schools selected to take part in the pilot
- Consultation with schools and external agencies regarding the pilot
- Implementation of the pilot from September 2007
- Tracking and ongoing development of the project (September 2007–July 2008)
- Initial findings from pilot (August 2008)
- Plans for the next stage

Questionnaire and data: initial findings

Before the intervention

- Attitudes and perception to sex and relationships are almost exactly the same when compared to different socio-economic backgrounds

- Young people have very clear ideas on who should be their main source of information on sex and relationships
- The majority of young people do not have sex under the age of 16
- Of the young people who do have sex under 16, 50 per cent or more were under the influence of alcohol
- The majority of young people think a steady relationship is more than eight weeks
- ALL overestimate how many peers they think are sexually active
- Their perception does not necessarily reflect their attitude
- Year 9 is the optimum time for the 'intervention', as this is the time when young people are developing their identity
- The majority of young people think it is OK to have sex under 16 IF in a steady relationship (over eight weeks)
- On delivery of SRE no one 'type' of person is favoured
- The skills, knowledge, confidence and relationship the facilitator has with young people is key

After the intervention

- The numbers of young people responding to 'it's OK to have sex under 16 if in a steady relationship' goes up in both Years 9 and 10
- There is a positive increase in per cent responding to the need to use more than one method of contraception
- No one size fits all ways of delivering SRE to young people
- Consultation of young people is key to the development of effective SRE programmes and messages
- Misperceptions still remain showing a need for ongoing high-quality SRE
- Partnerships between schools and specialist agencies play a key role in helping young people make healthy choices and reducing risky behaviour
- Further development is required in providing young people with a varied and high-quality SRE programme
- Further consultation, advice and guidance are required to develop the work and resources in and for schools

Examples of social norms messages used in schools

- *Don't believe everything they say!* Of Year 9 students, 96 per cent have not had sexual intercourse

- *You can wait a bit longer.* The majority of Year 9 students think you should wait until you are over 16 before having sex, even if you are in a steady relationship

- *How long is long?* Of Year 9 students 7 out of 10 think a steady relationship is more than eight weeks

- *Well worth the wait?* The majority of our students believe you should wait until you are over 16 to have sex

- *Safe sex is best.* Always use a condom

- *Don't believe everything you hear.* Statistics show 96 per cent of 14-year-olds have not had sex

- *They've done it all before.* The majority of Year 9 students think parents should be the main source of information about sex and relationships.

Examples of messages which are not so useful

- 93 per cent of students have not had sex under the influence of alcohol

- Over 85 per cent of students have not had sex

- 84 per cent of Year 9 students have never smoked a cigarette

- 76 per cent of all students think using tobacco is never a good thing to do

Challenges for schools

- Keeping to the timescale of the project

- Internet access

- Lack of parental support at evenings arranged to support the project

- Completing the second questionnaire with the same number of students

- Multi-agency availability to support the PSHE programme

- Development of resources

- Support by the school for the member of staff coordinating the project

- Fully involving students in the project

Ten Top Tips for Using the Social Norms approach in Schools.

1. Allow plenty of time for the project. At least two years including time allowed within each year you run the project.

2. Select up to three schools from a range of catchment areas to keep the project manageable (depending on how large your team is.)

3. Be prepared for schools not to meet your deadlines.

4. Support schools as much as possible to keep them on track.

5. Encourage schools to look at the social norms work as whole school focus not just PSHE. Sell it to Headteachers and senior management teams. Mention Every Child Matters, Ofsted, National Healthy Schools Status and the importance of consulting with young people.

6. Involve young people at the very beginning. They need to know why they are doing the questionnaire especially as they have to complete it twice. They are key to the development of the messages.

7. Be flexible and sympathetic to the needs of the school. (Things happen beyond their control sometimes.)

8. Involve external agencies to support and add value to the programme.

9. Allow a budget of up to £10,000 to support the development of the work.

10. Believe in the concept and be passionate about it. If you do so will others around you.

Next steps: the future for this project

- Broaden the project to include other counties interested in introducing the social norms approach

- Write a quick guide to analysing data and a programme for schools and other users

- Increase participation of schools in the project

- Extend the project to include two specific pieces of work on alcohol and sex and relationships in two upper schools and involve external agencies, parents, extended schools and Integrated Youth Support Services (IYSS) where possible

- Develop generic materials to support the normative messages

- Include the wider community to develop the campaign

- Ensure cohesion of current initiatives in schools of 'normative and delay approach'

- Seek additional funding to help support the project

- Engage young people in the consultation process using peer support from student consultants to ensure further impact on young people's choices
- Consolidate and expand messages by developing partnerships within the wider community
- Strengthen links to health services and offer one-to-one support and advice

Workshop 2: Rude, crude and socially unacceptable. Young people and pornography

Mark Limmer, Deputy Regional Teenage Pregnancy Coordinator, Government Office North West

Mark.Limmer@dh.gsi.gov.uk

The last few years have seen an increase in concern about the growing availability of pornography, its use and its impact in relation to young people, particularly young men. Despite this concern among those working directly with young people there has been very little research carried out in the UK in relation to pornography to match the growing literature in Scandinavia, the Netherlands and Canada.

This workshop provided an overview of the available research evidence, including studies on sexuality and sexual risk-taking among young people in Rochdale. Participants explored the patterns of pornography use among these young people, discussed evidence of an impact on their attitudes and behaviours and drew some conclusions as to how the issues can best be addressed from a policy perspective.

What is pornography?

The literal meaning of the word pornography is 'writing about harlots', although more recently it has come to be a catch-all description of obscene writings and images produced to 'elicit sexual arousal'. The important point is not so much to define pornography as to draw a distinction between it and 'erotica'. Conflating the two, as often happens, leads to circular arguments and a lack of clarity. For this workshop, I am defining pornography in terms of explicit materials which depict sexual activity in ways where there are clearly unequal power relationships. The enjoyment of nudity and erotica that depicts sexuality in terms of consensuality and equality seems relatively unproblematic – what turns this into pornography is exploitation and the abuse of power. What concerns us here is material that objectifies women and places them in a subordinate sexual role to men and which maintains and reflects masculine status and privilege in the sexual context. For this reason the workshop does not reflect on gay or feminist lesbian pornography.

Who is using pornography and where?

Among young men the use of pornography appears to be a majority activity: 98 per cent in a recent Swedish study (Haggstrom-Nordin and others 2005) and 87 per cent in a United States study (Carroll and others 2008). These same studies reported lower use among young women: 72 per cent and 31 per cent respectively. In the qualitative data from Rochdale, use of pornography was widespread among the young men but not reported often by the young women unless they were consuming it with male partners, with the implication that it was for the young man's pleasure not their own. Frequency of usage among the young men was difficult to gauge, but it was striking that they were all familiar with pornography, where to access it and what it contained – regardless of whether they reported consumption in their own lives. Pornography was accessed through a number of media, with the internet, DVD and mobile phones being the most often reported, and whilst there was evidence of the sharing of pornography and discussion of what was available with each other, there was little reporting of shared watching of pornography beyond short clips on mobile phones. Pornography was essentially viewed in private, and the access points enabled this privacy in ways that the historical necessity to purchase publicly precluded. Many of the young men had access to computers, usually in their bedrooms, and so had access to internet pornography that they could download and share privately. Pornography use seems to hold a paradoxically public and private position in these young men's lives – the majority acknowledged accessing pornography, it was a source of discussion, but it was essentially consumed in private.

What are they watching – the 'pornographic discourses'

Whilst there was a significant range of pornographic material being watched, from the hardcore, extreme and excessively explicit end to the more late-night Channel Five, MTV, 'softer end', there are discourses that run through all the pornography that is being consumed and the constant reinforcement of these discourses has a profound impact on the sexual attitudes of both young men and women. The fact that some of the discourses clearly resonate with societal beliefs about sexual roles and gender power relations gives them an increased sense of validity and their repetition further cements them into place. The tendency to focus concern on the more extreme end of pornography misses the point, which is that it is the constant reinforcement of unequal gender sexual relationships that runs through more 'mainstream' pornography that is influencing most young people and that this contributes to their understanding of the appropriate ways of expressing their sexuality.

From the reports of the pornography that young people were accessing and from their discussions with each other within the research, six key discourses emerge that are consistent regardless of whether the material was considered 'hard' or 'soft'. The first is that sex is a physical experience that takes place within an emotional vacuum; it is the physicality – culminating in male ejaculation – that is important, with little concern for context or feelings. The second discourse is one of compulsory heterosexuality, for men at least. Whilst there is a significant amount of gay pornography available, this was outside what the young people involved in these research projects saw as appropriate and they made no reference to it. The exception was lesbianism, which plays a large part in the reported pornography usage of the young men and which was seen as acceptable. This reflects the approved sexualised masculine discourse that requires young men to be heterosexual and which normalises homophobia – but as lesbianism lies outside that discourse it can be incorporated into male fantasy and pornography. Leading on from this, the third discourse reflects that it is men who are the target for pornography and consequently it privileges men's experience over women's. Intercourse and male ejaculation signal the climax and completion of the act – it is these that are the point of sex. The fourth discourse demands that men should take the lead in, and be in control of, sex. and to do this requires the right equipment and the right performance. The ideal, reflected by pornography, demands that the man is good at sex, he has a large penis, that neither lets him down through failing to erect nor through ejaculating too soon, and that he never refuses a sexual opportunity. The fifth discourse positions women as always willing to have sex – even if at first they don't realise it. The proficiency of the male performance will inevitably induce pleasure and orgasm. In this discourse the pleasure that the woman takes from sex reflects not on her, but on the expertise and artistry of the man – her sexual pleasure is his achievement. The final discourse is that there are no negative consequences to sex – no regret afterwards, no pregnancy and no infections – and in this no-consequence arena there is clearly no need for condom use, nor any discussion or negotiation.

The fact that these discourses are both near universal to the pornography that the young people reported, and that they so closely reflect the ways that gendered sexuality is played out in society – albeit in an isolated and extreme form – means that they have a validity; they affirm a stereotyped and unequal sexual context. As will be explored in the next section, there is some evidence from these cohorts that suggests that these discourses inherent in pornography impact on the behaviour and attitudes of both young men and young women.

What is the impact of pornography?

Identifying direct causal relationships between the use of pornography and changes to sexual attitudes and behaviours is difficult, although some recent studies from Sweden (Tyden and Rogala 2004; Haggstrom-Nordin and others 2005), the Netherlands (Peter and Valkenburg 2006, 2007) and the United States (Carroll and others 2008) have highlighted some of the key associations and appear to demonstrate convincingly some impact to exposure to pornography. The impact demonstrated included changes in attitudes and in behaviours, and although equivalent research has not been carried out in the UK, there is no reason to expect that the results would differ significantly.

In the data from the studies in Rochdale the focus was more on the discourses that underpinned behaviour and on young people's reported impact from their own or their sexual partner's consumption of pornography. The reported impact of pornography was clearly gendered, with young women significantly more likely to see it as problematic and being able to identify how it had impacted negatively on their sexual relationships. The impact from their perspective was mainly that pornography created expectations in relation to their availability and to the sexual activities they would be expected to perform. Whilst most of the young women felt that they could resist the pressures, they also resented the fact that they had to:

> They get really sick ideas from watching it [pornography] and if you don't do them then they moan.
>
> (Young woman aged 16)

They saw pornography as creating expectations of them that they were both unable and unwilling to fulfil and they also recognised the impact on young men who had been led to have high expectations of their own experience that were also unfulfilled.

> That [pornography] is why they think that sex is supposed to be so amazing to them, and then they're disappointed ... and the girl's disappointed because the lad's crap.
>
> (Young woman aged 17)

The consequence of the young man's sense of failed performance has repercussions for the young woman as Holland and others (1994) make clear in their description of how young women are made to be the scapegoat and cause of sexual failure to deflect from the potential vulnerability of the young man. Young women also saw pornography as depicting sex in a way that was distant from what they wanted to experience; they expressed the desire for 'someone to give me cuddles and listen to me' and for sex to be a reflection of something deeper and more based around emotion. This wasn't a polarisation that positioned young women as the antithesis of sex for pleasure and fun, but rather that they felt somehow outside of the sexual encounter, that the young men thought of sex as being for themselves rather than a shared experience – a discourse which runs throughout pornography.

The impact of pornography on the young men involved in the studies was much more clearly articulated: '[it] makes you want to try new things – take it up a notch'. That is not to say that they saw pornography as reality; they were able to recognise that this was not sex as it was, or could be for them. So the impact was less a sense of copying what they had seen and more a validation of behaviours and activities that were already a part of their self-perception as men. The discourses inherent in pornography that were discussed earlier were resonant of their sexualised masculinity – pornography provides a blueprint for the idealised sexual male, not a manual. It is this validation of sexualised masculinity that provides some of the power that pornography has in shaping young men's attitudes and behaviours with its compulsory heterosexuality, its emphasis on sexual performance and expertise, its privileging of male pleasure and its reinforcement of young men as sexual beings. Young men were able to say that they understood that pornography wasn't real – 'that's just fantasy sex that, innit' – and that in some cases that they felt it was 'hanging' or 'disgusting'; but it was clear that despite their protestations it did have an influence through its discourses that reassured them that their position as the privileged sexual gender was still in place.

The downside for young men in relation to pornography is that it can create expectations that they can never fulfil – they almost certainly haven't got huge penises, they can't delay ejaculation indefinitely and their partners will not always achieve multiple orgasms – and consequently they feel like sexual failures. For most young men this is less of a problem because they have alternative sexual influences through families, schools, peers and other sections of the media. However, for some young men this is problematic, because although they are not simply passive consumers of pornography and they can critique what they have seen, to do so requires them to access an alternative frame of reference. For some young men, and in these studies it was those who were most socially excluded, disengaged and powerless, there was no other frame of reference that could effectively challenge and counterbalance the influence of pornography. In short, one of the few ways available to them to express masculinity is through sex, and the approved sexual expression of masculinity is encapsulated in pornography. More, there is no alternative frame of reference provided by fathers, institutions or peers to give a counterbalance. It is these young men who are most immediately impacted on by pornography, but ultimately – and to varying degrees – by reinforcing dominant male sexual discourses, pornography impacts on all young men and all young women.

Why do young people use pornography?

In the data collected in these studies young women rarely talked of accessing pornography in their own right – those that did watch pornography tended to do so with a partner and were at best ambivalent and more often hostile to it and the impact it had on young men. So this section will principally reflect on why young men say that they use pornography. Whilst the young men would admit and discuss that they enjoyed pornography, most were reluctant to admit either that they derived pleasure and used it for masturbation, or that they learned anything from it, although there were exceptions, particularly in relation to the latter. Admitting, as a young man, that you use pornography for the purposes of masturbation is problematic in two ways. Firstly, masturbation, remarkably, remains a taboo subject in the UK (although not always; see below) and the self-image of sitting masturbating in front of the internet is not one that young men are eager to portray to each other. Secondly, approved masculinity requires that young men's sexual needs are met through sex with young women, so although there is a tacit acceptance of masturbation, it is rarely expressed as a positive expression of masculine sexuality. Despite these preclusions to reporting, it was clear that pornography and masturbation played a significant role in young men's developing sexuality, in a way that it has throughout history.

In terms of reported learning from pornography there were two distinct discourses – the first denied it on the basis that not only did the young men already know the information – admitting ignorance of sexual matters is in itself problematic – but also that pornography wasn't for that purpose. As one young man put it

You don't go 'I want to learn about sex, I'll get a porn film'. It's like 'I want a wank, I'll watch a porn film'. That's more like it.

(Young man aged 17)

On the other hand there were a significant number of young men who said that they used pornography to learn more about sex, and that the reason they did so was because sex education failed to teach them what they wanted to know. Often it came too late. But the main criticism was that it failed to show how to have sex, how to arouse a woman, what everything looks like – in reality rather than in pictures. The irony is that young men, in a perfectly reasonable attempt to access information and images that reflect the reality of sex, end up accessing sites that provide explicitness but within a distorted context. The intense need to be able to perform sex, to not look foolish and ignorant in front of peers and to know how to take the lead in sex, all of which are essential elements of a young men's sexualised masculinity, turn them towards pornography. The lack of alternative sources of explicit, young men orientated but balanced images of sex and sexuality creates genuine problems and is an indictment of the quality of sexual health education provision within and outside of schools.

Finally, using and discussing heterosexual pornography provides young men with a way of demonstrating their own heterosexuality and serves to place other sexualities outside the accepted norm. Homophobia and the active demonstration of not being gay is hugely powerful in the development of young masculinities – see for example the work of Debbie Epstein (Epstein and Johnson 1998) and Emma Renold (2003) – and in lieu of demonstrating this through active sexual relations with women, pornography provides a valuable standby. In the same way, pornography clearly positions women in the subordinate sexual role, allowing young men a proxy demonstration of their masculinity.

Conclusion

Pornography is everywhere. It is accessible through a wide range of media and affects all young people, male and female. The discussion has shifted now to how do we deal with its presence and how do we enable young people to make sense of it, to see it for what it is and to avoid defining their sexual lives in relation to it? Clearly pornography has an impact, and an impact that is gendered. There is a need to address the impact on young men and young women differently. For young women pornography creates a sexual environment where they are subordinate, where their sexual health is put at risk and where their own sexual pleasures are made secondary to those of young men. For young men the situation is paradoxical; on the one hand pornography reflects and preserves their superior sexual status in relation to women, and on the other it creates expectations of them that they cannot fulfil and which distort their relationships with young women. For young gay men, mainstream pornography simply marginalises and subordinates their sexuality, creating fertile ground for homophobia. On a more positive note, most young people navigate their way through, they have alternative frames of reference that support and bolster healthier images of themselves and their sexuality, but there remains a need for all those that are concerned about the good emotional and physical sexual health of young people to actively and explicitly address pornography and its impact.

Discussion

Following the presentation, the workshop participants discussed the following issues.

- Most of the participants had some experience of working with young people who had been exposed to pornography. This was reflected in the young people's use of language. Some were very young when they were first exposed.

- The question was posed that if everybody was well informed about sex, would pornography have less impact on sexual behaviour? Concern about pornography may not just be about sex; it is also about power, exploitation and the reinforcement of a gender imbalance. If young people have other frames of reference they could challenge what they see. However, despite this, it may be similar to how we view images in magazines. We know that images of women in magazines have been airbrushed or manipulated and we know they are not real, but we may still look at magazines and think, 'I wish I looked like that'.

- There is little research looking at whether people watching pornography have empathy for the people in it, but some of the language that young people use (for example, 'sluts') may reflect their views on the 'actors'.

- Consumer figures on pornography are difficult to establish as much of the porn is free to view on the internet. There has also been a rise in the use of mobile phones with cameras to make and distribute porn. Images can be passed around, for example in a school, very quickly and have a damaging affect on those in the image (who may not have realised what they were involved in).

- Internet safety is an increasing concern. Porn 'pop-ups' are common and difficult to control. Software is available to control this but this is not highly publicised.

- Mainstream pornography does not provide positive images around gender, sexual orientation, race or disability.

- Young people are very interested in the details around sex: the most frequently asked question was: 'How do we know we're doing it right?'

- Teacher training on this subject is a challenge. It needs a very competent and confident educator to talk about pornography and sexual needs in SRE. Despite young people's questions there is reluctance to go into this in any depth. Youth workers may be better positioned to approach this issue. Also they work with smaller groups in less formal settings.

- There is a need for more research, but doing research on this topic may be culturally challenging in the UK compared to, for example, Sweden, where asking young people intimate questions is not considered problematic. We need to create a context in which we can have these conversations.

Workshop 3: Parents – building bridges between parents and schools

David Kesterton, project manager, Speakeasy, fpa
davidk@fpa.org.uk

To ensure that SRE messages are consistent and parents feel supported and confident to talk to their children, it is vital that parents and schools can work together on this topic. The Children's Plan sets out new requirements for schools to engage with parents and SRE is a topic where many parents would like support. The following workshop provided an example of a project which works to build parents' confidence, and invited participants to explore ways in which schools can support parents.

Ten of the most common questions from Speakeasy parents

- How do I start talking about sex and relationships?
- How can I get over feeling embarrassed?
- What if my child knows more than I do?
- At what age should I start talking about sex?
- How do I ensure they understand my values?
- What about peer pressure and sex in the media?
- Will talking about it encourage sexual activity?
- My child might be gay. What should I do?
- Don't they get sex education at school?
- How do I keep my child safe online?

Speakeasy – the need to support parents to talk with their children

'Children are growing up younger'
'The pressures are greater'
'Children want to learn from us'
'I feel embarrassed and awkward in talking about sex'
'We can't leave it all to the schools'

'Children whose parents talk to them about sexual matters and provide sexuality education at home are more likely than others to postpone sexual activity'
(Blake and others, 2001)

The way sexual issues are discussed with children is as important as what is said, for example discussing issues rather than dictating behaviour. If parents are able to discuss sexual matters with their children in a skilled and comfortable manner, it may help their children to discuss sex with their partners.
(NHS Health Development Agency, 2001)

Aims of Speakeasy

- To enable parents to talk to their children about sex and relationships

- To increase parents' factual knowledge about sex and relationships

- To increase parents' confidence and communication skills about sex and relationships

- To provide a step towards learning/personal development for parents in priority groups

- To support parenting practitioners in using the Speakeasy model in their work

Learning outcomes

- Physical and emotional changes at puberty

- SRE in the context of family life

- Responding to the needs of children in relation to sex and relationships in the context of family life

- Social and cultural attitudes towards sex and sexuality as they relate to children

- Methods of contraception

- Sexually transmitted infections and safer sex

- Strategies for keeping children safe from harm

- SRE in schools taking account of statutory and non-statutory guidance

What parents reported – an evaluation

	Before course	After course	Change
Confidence	2.99	4.4	47%
Knowledge area			
Puberty	3.02	4.44	47%
STIs	2.59	4.33	67%
Contraception	3.3	4.56	38%
Keeping safe	3.37	4.56	35%

Parents rated themselves, using a scale of one to five, on their knowledge before and after the course.

Parental reactions to school-based sessions

'I was surprised at how little of the SRE policy was statutory. This seems to give schools very vague guidance as to what should be taught in school.'

'I was surprised that I was unable to get the SRE policy from any of my daughters' schools. The secondary school did not even know that there was one.'

'I think parents should attend some kind of group to understand [the school's view] and for them to hear why SRE should be taught.'

'Parents are not mentioned – I was appalled'

'After being on the course I realise how much is still 'presumed' to be the parents' responsibility (rightly so) by the Department for Children, Schools and Families and how much, as a parent, I presume is being taught in school. We should work together.'

Bridging school/home – people to consider

Head
PSHE lead
Governors inc. parent governors
Parent Teacher Associations (PTAs)
SRE advisor
Healthy Schools
Teenage Pregnancy

Bridging school/home – people involved

Parent support advisors
Family Liaison staff
Family Information Projects
Home School Partnership
Parent champions for SRE development

Discussion

Following the presentation the participants discussed the following questions.

- How to create a sense of partnership on SRE between school and home

- How to reassure parents who express concern about SRE

- Beginning to reach hard to engage parents

The following is a summary of the discussion.

- Schools are aware they need to engage parents in the formation of their SRE policies to gain their school Healthy Schools accreditation and so many schools have a community classroom or some other venue that's appropriate for doing the work.

- Schools need to move from solely providing information to parents on what they will be covering to actively helping them to speak to their children.

- Parents report enjoying working with other parents.

- Parent groups help them build their confidence.

- Having a taster session can encourage parents to try it out without having to make an immediate commitment.

- The format of Speakeasy can also be used to introduce other topics like drugs and alcohol.

- Parents may also need help on topics like sexual orientation if their child is gay. Schools have a role in providing parents with information on these topics as well as signposting to local support groups.

- It may be helpful if SRE changed its name to put the focus on 'relationships', especially in primary schools. This would make parents less nervous about the topic.

- The debate (in the media at least) is that it is the parents rather than the school's responsibility to teach SRE, but many parents expect schools to be teaching it. They are often surprised at how little is actually taught – the end result being that children are not learning anything from reliable sources, but are relying on their friends and the media.

- Parents appreciate being able to borrow resources such as DVDs and story books from schools to help them with SRE at home.

- In order to get a commitment from schools to do parenting work they will need specific funding. There is also a need to look at existing levers, for example extended schools work.

- It is important to highlight that the information provided in projects like Speakeasy is factual and does not promote any type of lifestyle or pregnancy option.

Handy Guide for Parents and Carers in Hertfordshire

Parents are often used as an excuse: 'Parents won't like it'. But, in the experience of Speakeasy, parents appreciate the opportunity to get involved and to know what the schools are teaching in SRE. In Hertfordshire, a leaflet was produced for parents on this topic which was well received (Herts TP Partnership, 2008).

Key topics covered in the leaflet.

- What exactly is SRE?

- What does SRE involve?

- How do schools deliver SRE?

- Why is SRE so important?

- Why worry?

- Young people's views

- How does SRE help?

- What is our county's goal?

- How is SRE taught?

- What are my rights?

- Where can I get further information?

Taken from Herts TP Partnership www.hertsdirect.org/yrccouncil

---

Workshop 4: Involving young people – using the 'Are You Getting It Right?' Pupil Audit Toolkit to consult young people on SRE

Lesley de Meza, co-author of the Toolkit, PSHE education
consultant, trainer and writer
lesley@lesleydemeza.com

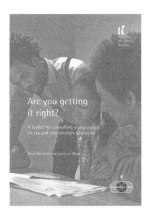

The aim of this workshop was to provide an overview of SEF's Toolkit to help schools consult with young people on SRE. Participants looked at why SRE is important in the context of the new Personal Well-being Programme of Study, why it is essential we audit SRE provision and why young people should be involved in this process. Participants also had the opportunity to think about how they would use the Toolkit in their local areas.

Why is SRE in schools important?

In the new national curriculum for secondary schools, PSHE has become 'PSHE education'. It has two new Programmes of Study (PoS): 'Personal Well-being' and 'Economic Well-being and Financial Capability'. SRE is taught within Personal Well-being.

Personal well-being

... helps young people embrace change, feel positive about who they are and enjoy healthy, safe, responsible and fulfilled lives ... recognise and manage risk, take increasing responsibility for themselves, their choices and behaviours and make positive contributions.

...explore similarities and differences ... discuss social and moral dilemmas ... learn to deal with challenges and accommodate diversity in all its forms.

...reflect on and clarify values and attitudes ... identify and articulate feelings and emotions ... form and maintain relationships.

Key learning processes

The key learning processes in PSHE education include:

- Critical reflection
- Decision-making and managing risk
- Developing relationships and working with others
- Self-development
- Exploration
- Enterprise
- Financial capability

Range and content

The range and content which are relevant to SRE include:

- *Personal identities* – personal and social values, targets and goal setting
- *Healthy lifestyles* – sexual health, drugs, nutrition, physical and emotional changes
- *Risk* – understanding risk, basic knowledge of first aid
- *Relationships* – different types of relationship, roles and responsibilities of parents/ carers
- *Diversity* – similarities, differences and diversity among people from different races, culture, ability/disability, gender, age and sexual orientation and the impact of prejudice, bullying and discrimination

The learning experience

What would make SRE a more 'compelling learning experience' for young people?

- More than biology
- Being part of PSHE education

- Not a 'one-off' intervention
- Addressing knowledge, attitudes and skills
- Active learning, for example drama, role-play, discussion, etc.
- Being relevant to the young people's needs/wants

What young people say about SRE

- There is a big gap between, what young people need and what they get
- It doesn't meet the needs of young people
- Too late, not relevant, not enough, too biological, too boring

(UKYP 2007; SEF 2008)

Why should we audit/review SRE?

- Window of opportunity to improve SRE
- Recommendation in the national SRE Review
- Schools' statutory duty to well-being
- New secondary curriculum – 'Personal Well-being'
- Primary curriculum under review
- Public health concerns: teenage pregnancy, STI rates, etc.

Why should we consult young people?

- They know what they need
- To be able to differentiate learning
- It ensures their 'buy-in' and engagement
- To ensure the teaching style is appropriate for the topic

How is an audit cycle carried out?

- Preparation – identify an auditing team
- Step 1 – Identify how good SRE fits with local priorities
- Step 2 – Review the existing policy and curriculum

- Step 3 – Identify what stakeholders want from SRE

- Step 4 – Ensure that you include young people (as stakeholders)

- Step 5 – In consultation, draft new policy and curriculum

What is the SRE Pupil Audit Toolkit?

The Toolkit is a set of simple structured activities that allows young people to reflect on their SRE, identify gaps and recommend improvements.

What are the activities?

Activity 1:   Setting ground rules

Activity 2:   Taking stock of current SRE

Activities 3 and 4: Identifying gaps in existing provision

Activity 5:   Exploring values underpinning SRE

Activity 6:   Assessing needs

Activity 7:   Reflection and recommendations to improve SRE

How to encourage schools to audit/review SRE and use the Toolkit

Schools should be encouraged to consult with pupils and use the audit toolkit because it is a criteria for the National Healthy School Standard and it contributes the five Every Child Matters outcomes as measured by Ofsted. Consultation is also required on Ofsted's schools self-evaluation form and it forms part of CPD-PSHE evidence demonstrating the impact on schools. The consultation process forms part of the citizenship aspect of PSHE education.

Discussion

After the presentation, participants discussed the following questions:

- What actions can you take to start the process of reviewing SRE and ensuring your young people have a voice?

- Who needs to be involved, how do you get it on the agenda and what are the possible challenges?

Participants discussed the Toolkit and its applicability and the following issues arose:

- Need to ensure a balance between having the flexibility to design a curriculum based on the needs of your pupils and having sample curricula ready to support teachers

- Consulting with young people is a powerful tool, but unless they can see the changes their views have made it becomes meaningless

- Young people enjoy doing 'research' – in one school the Year 11 pupils enjoyed preparing games and resources for the Year 7s to use and researching what the Year 7s needed

- There are enough 'levers' to make people feel 'Here's another thing we're being forced to do'. It's about winning hearts and minds. It's got to be about actually getting people to feel we want to consult with young people because it's worthwhile, because it's going to produce outcomes that we actually want and value

- A large number of local authorities are now basing their strategies on Every Child Matters outcomes and that in itself acts as a lever

Workshop 5: Faith and Values – exploring SRE in a multi-faith society looking at local case studies

Sarah Thistle, Change for Children Manager, VTE&S
sarah.thistle@vtplc.com

Hansa Patel-Kanwal (OBE), Independent Consultant and Life Member of SEF
strategicchoices@yahoo.com

Work around Faith and Values and SRE is about embarking on a perpetual journey because we are dealing with constantly evolving, dynamic issues and communities. The aim of this workshop was to enable participants to explore issues around Faith and Values and SRE and share emerging best practice. This session provided signposting to further information and support. It was designed either as a refresher session or to raise awareness of these issues.

A case study: Waltham Forest

Excellent work with faith communities to explore a single faith and values framework to inform sex and relationships work is contributing to community cohesion.

(Ofsted 2008)

Background

The School Improvement Service in Waltham Forest is committed to ensuring that every pupil in the borough receives their entitlement to high-quality SRE. With such a richly diverse community, we recognised the importance of developing a local values framework with faith leaders that could both underpin a school's SRE programme and demonstrate multi-faith support for the work in our schools.

The Change for Children Team, supported by Waltham Forest Primary Care Trust (PCT), invited members of SACRE, the Standing Advisory Council on Religious Education, and other faith representatives involved directly in SRE delivery, to work together to develop a consensus around the values that should underpin this critical aspect of young people's education.

Process

Following discussion with SACRE members, it was agreed to convene two facilitated evening workshops to draft the values' framework. These were planned a month apart, to provide the group with thinking time as well as an opportunity to consult with their faith communities between workshops.

The Change for Children Team commissioned Hansa Patel-Kanwal, who had worked on the national Faith and Values and SRE project, to lead the facilitation of the workshops in partnership with the team.

At the beginning of the first session the group acknowledged that there would be different views and beliefs, relating to some of the issues for discussion, and identified the importance of establishing a 'working together agreement' to ensure a safe, supportive and effective working environment for everyone. The group agreement was:

- Please respect the need for confidentiality

- Please respect each other's right to hold different opinions, attitudes and beliefs

- We encourage respectful disagreement and challenge

- Try to be specific and own your perspective by using 'I' statements

- Please explain any jargon

- Please participate as fully as possible and support the participation of others

- Please try to enjoy listening, hearing, thinking and clarifying

Workshop A

Participants were given an overview of national guidance on school-based SRE. They were invited to work together in pairs or small groups to clarify with each other what their particular faith has to say about various sex and relationship issues. Although there were some differences, there was a large degree of consensus across the faith perspectives. The whole group then discussed, and attempted to reach consensus on, the values that they felt underpinned effective SRE.

Following Workshop A, notes of the whole group discussion were distilled into a set of draft values statements and circulated to the group. Members were asked to confirm whether these statements were a true reflection of the consensus that had been reached at the workshop and invited to offer feedback in advance or at the next workshop.

Workshop B

Participants worked together to refine the statements and then action planned how the consultation would be opened up to their wider faith communities.

Following wider consultation, the amended statements were brought back to a SACRE meeting for final agreement by the whole membership.

Outcomes

- Increased understanding of the content and need for SRE amongst faith leaders
- Increased support for SRE, based on a shared values framework
- Increased understanding across faith groups of the different and similar faith perspectives relating to sex and relationships

Next steps

The values framework for SRE will be launched at an event for schools in early 2009. Schools will be encouraged to actively sign up to the framework. SACRE members agreed to be a point of contact for schools with queries about faith perspectives relating to SRE issues. The School Improvement Service will act as a conduit for these enquiries.

Discussion

The participants were encouraged to discuss the following questions.

What work have you developed/are you developing around faith, values and SRE?

Participants discussed a range of projects which involve faith communities including using the following:

- No Outsiders (focusing on homophobia)
- Christopher Winter Project (primary schools)
- Working with the local mosques
- Training for parents and governors
- Inter-faith forums
- Linking sports to sexual health screening
- A women's heath group for Muslim women with a focus on body image to make SRE easier to introduce

Identify one issue you have encountered in your work around Faith and Values and SRE.

Issues that participants encountered included the following:

- Teachers at the start of the SRE project expressed concerns about the reaction of parents of a particular faith, however, despite these concerns, hardly any children are withdrawn from primary SRE

- Parents are frequently used as an excuse for not teaching SRE: 'Parents won't like it'.

- Pregnant girls are still being excluded from some faith schools

- The perception that there is an overemphasis on sex in SRE and the need for a name change which puts 'relationships' first

- The challenge to make sure SRE is relevant to all pupils regardless of faith

Some of the solutions discussed included the following.

- The importance of involving stakeholders from the beginning of the process

- Not making the assumption that everybody from the same faith holds the same views regarding sex, relationships and sexual health

- Headteachers and senior leadership teams need to champion SRE

- The need to do preparatory work with all staff and parents before starting work in class

- Not just focusing on schools but developing training programmes for faith leaders

London Borough of Waltham Forest
Values Framework for Sex & Relationship Education (SRE)

1. Relationship education is at the core of SRE and is the vehicle through which teaching about sex will be delivered.

2. Children and young people need to be at the heart of the messages we provide through SRE by ensuring their health and well-being are promoted and maintained.

3. Within a whole school approach, SRE will be age appropriate and be provided according to children and young people's level of understanding. It will equip children and young people with life skills such as negotiating and asserting themselves within all their relationships.

4. To develop a critical awareness, SRE should address and challenge irresponsible messages from the media in discussions with children and young people.

5. SRE should empower, enable, encourage and support young people to make sense of conflicting messages and resist peer pressure so they can make informed decisions about their personal relationships.

6. Information should be provided in a consistent way by confident educators, and other relevant professionals, who are trained in line with national guidance (e.g. Ofsted, DCSF & QCA) and are respectful of different faith and cultural perspectives.

7. SRE should encourage children and young people to explore each other's faith and cultural perspectives in an objective and respectful way.

8. SRE should be informed by an awareness of the context within which our children and young people are living.

9. SRE should ensure that children and young people have opportunities to express their views appropriately in safe and supportive environments within schools and other community based settings.

10. To avoid confusion, SRE should explore where there are differences and overlaps between faith perspectives and cultural views on specific issues within the curriculum.

11. Parents and carers have a key role in SRE and particularly in clarifying their faith and cultural perspectives on relationships and sex. Therefore, schools, families and local communities need to work in partnership to support children and young people through their physical, emotional and spiritual development.

12. To encourage young people to develop mutually respectful relationships, SRE should discuss how they can keep themselves and others safe. They need to understand that all rights have responsibilities and all actions have consequences.

13. To encourage young people to develop into responsible adults who can maintain their health and well-being, SRE includes providing information about local and national sexual health services.

14. To ensure that children and young people understand the law, SRE needs to address the legislation around sex and relationships and discuss potential conflicts with their faith or cultural perspectives in an objective manner.

15. SRE needs to help children and young people to recognise that prejudice, discrimination and bullying are harmful and unacceptable to all our faith principles.

16. Within the context of mutually respectful relationships, young people should understand that sexual intimacy involves strong emotions and should involve a sense of respect for one's own and others' feelings, decisions and actions.

Workshop 6: 'Scored project' – working creatively, using football, to engage with vulnerable young people in SRE

Karina Bowkett
Michelle Thompson
Chris McCabe
The Young People's Health Project
Karina_Bowkett@birmingham.gov.uk

The aim of this workshop was to explore the award winning 'Scored project' (winner of the 2008 fpa Pamela Sheridan award), which used football training as a method to engage young people in SRE. Using sport in this way ensures that any work on sexual health starts where the young people 'are at' and uses language and concepts that they understand and can relate to. Using the analogy 'fair play' on and off the pitch helped to explore sexual relationships through questions like 'Are you fair when you're scoring a goal, or when you're scoring a girl?', 'Where do her rights come into it?' and 'Where do your rights come into it?'

Consultation and background

- Currently working in the area – consultation with young people, young people out of school, part-time timetables, isolation, high level of truanting

- Teenage Pregnancy Unit – identified Shard End as a priority area with one of the highest teenage pregnancy rates in Birmingham at 89 conceptions per 1000

- Demographics and associated risk factors – low socio-economic group, poor educational attainment and exclusion or risk of being excluded

- Poor SRE at school

The area – Shard End, East Birmingham

- Shard End ward has one of the lowest school attendance and attainment rates in Birmingham East and North PCT, with twice as many children obtaining 5 GCSEs in Sutton Vesey and Sutton Four Oaks as in Shard End
- Shard End is in the top 5 per cent of deprived wards in England and ranks fifth in the country for low educational attainment

Aims and objectives

National aims

- To halve the under-18 conception rate by 2010
- To establish a firm downward trend in the under-16 rate
- To increase the proportion of teenage parents in education, training or employment to 60 per cent by 2010
- To reduce their risk of long-term social exclusion

What we hope to achieve locally

The project aims to raise awareness among young men about the responsibilities of engaging in a sexual relationship, safe sex, the consequences of unprotected sex and the role, responsibilities and rights of fatherhood.

- Facts and function
- Contraception/protection
- Pregnancy and parenting
- Relationships
- Future choices

Why the connection between SRE and football?

- What the young people wanted to do
- Engaging and retaining the interest of young men by providing one-hour football training
- Using practical-based delivery techniques
- Analogy of 'fair play' on and off the pitch
- Transferable skills – communication, negotiation, etc.
- Decision-making

- Team work

- Goal setting – aspiration for the future

- Yellow and red card system for behaviour on and off the pitch which supports creating a safe learning environment and set boundaries

Learning outcomes of the project

- Knowledge of sexual organs, awareness of the body and its different functions

- Knowledge of STIs, how they are transmitted, how they affect the body and how they can be tested for and treated

- Knowledge of local services providing sexual health advice and information, contraception services and testing for STIs

- Awareness of all the different types of contraception, their reliability, pros and cons, methods of use, what to do if the contraception fails and where to get emergency contraception

- Awareness of pressure and improved decision-making skills around sexual health situations and drug/alcohol situations

- Recognition of the complexities and responsibilities of parenting, the financial costs and the social stigma experienced by young parents

- An understanding and assessment of the impact having a child has on personal and social life, as well as educational and long-term achievements

- An opportunity for the young males to look after a reality baby

- Improved football skills

- Development of social and personal skills – team building, meeting new people and making friends

Activities

Each activity had a sexual health focus but related the principles back to football.

Example activities 1 – Know your bits

Why is it important to know your sexual organs and how they function? Why is it important to know the rules of football?

LEARNING OUTCOME: Knowledge of sexual organs, awareness of body and different functions

Using familiar objects to explain parts of the body

- Cream Eggs or Kinder Eggs – Ovaries
- Banana – Penis
- Plums – Testicles
- Liquorice Laces – Fallopian tubes
- Pear – Womb
- Condom – Vagina

The following are example of links between knowing your body and knowing the rules of football.

- So there's no fouling or unfair play
- You know if something's wrong
- To stay safe and not get hurt, both on the pitch and when having sex
- To understand the game rules, the rules of your body and how it functions and to know if something's wrong
- To acknowledge the enjoyment aspect and about having fun
- To feel confident about your body – being in control on the pitch, protecting yourself in a sexual relationship

Example activities 2 – Relationship pitch

Different types of relationships, based on the three different actions in football. Who do you defend, tackle and attack in a relationship? The importance of communication on and off the pitch

LEARNING OUTCOME: To be able to identify qualities and skills for a healthy relationship and identify pressuring situations and unacceptable relationships

The following is an example of a discussion around this activity.

If you 'attack' (are aggressive or angry towards) your friends what's bad about that? Are you able to support that friend if you're attacking them? How you defend your friends and look after them as well as be just good friends. What are the friendly aspects to friendship? How do you tackle problems in a relationship?

Example activities 3 – Protection on and off the pitch

How young people protect themselves on the pitch when playing football and off the pitch in a relationship

LEARNING OUTCOME: Awareness of all of the different types of contraception, their reliability, pros and cons, methods of use, what to do if the contraception fails and local services for young people

Achievement – accreditation

This project was accredited.

- Ten young people achieved the National Open College Network Level 1 – Improving own learning and performance
- Sixteen young people achieved the St John Ambulance/First Aid Certificate – Emergency Life Support for All Ages

Key themes to ensure success

- Consultation with young people
- Working creatively with where they are at
- Flexible approach – ability to adapt the programme
- Partnership work – Teenage Pregnancy Coordinator and PCT, school nurses, school library
- School nurses, schools, library
- 'Coachright' having a professional football coach
- Support from managers

Discussion

The participants asked questions relating to the project.

- **How the project was funded?**

Young People's Health Project is not mainstream funded so there is no specific budget for SRE work, however the Youth Service pays for staff. The Scored Project was funded by the Teenage Pregnancy Unit under the youth service development programmes. We are exploring ways of tapping into funds the Football Association may have.

- **The age range of the participants and whether it can be adapted for the younger age range?**

For age 13 and, yes, we could adapt the programme, especially the body parts and relationships aspects. We could also cover testicular cancer in future sessions.

How the programme was evaluated?

We used the accreditation as a measure. Also we evaluated it at the end of each session to find out what the participants had learned. On the first course we did a base line on what they knew and then we could evaluate what they then knew at the end. Trying to keep in with the football theme, they set goals for themselves and what they wanted to achieve by the end of the project, for example to achieve their First Aid or their Level 1 NOCN, improve their football or just to make new friends. Observation is a key thing to ensure whether the project is working.

Workshop 7: What works? 17 characteristics of effective sex education

Douglas Kirby, Senior Research Scientist, ETR Associates
dougk@etr.org

This workshop was a continuation from the presentation in the morning plenary session. It was an opportunity for participants to explore in more depth the characteristics of effective sex education that have been identified through research over the last 21 years. These 17 characteristics (see page 76) have been categorised into three components

- Category 1: Characteristics describing the process of development
- Category 2: Characteristics describing the curriculum content
- Category 3: Characteristics describing the implementation of the curriculum

Category 1: Characteristics describing the process of development

1. Involved multiple people with different experience and backgrounds to design curriculum

Topics covered were as follows:

- Theory
- Research on adolescent sexual behaviour
- Educational theory and curriculum design
- Experience teaching youth about sex
- Cultural knowledge
- Evaluation

2. Assessed relevant needs and assets of the target group

3. Used logic model approach

1. Specified the health goals (prevention of HIV, other STDs or pregnancy)
2. Specified the behaviours that cause or prevent HIV, other STDs or pregnancy
3. Used theory, research and personal experience to identify the psychosocial sexual risk and protective factors affecting those behaviours
4. Designed activities to affect those factors

Curriculum activities	Risk and protection factors	Important behaviours	Goals
Practise insisting on condom use in role-play	Increased self-efficacy to insist on condom use	Increased use of condoms	Reduced STDs/HIV and pregnancy
Identify 'safe' places to obtain condoms	Increased self-efficacy to obtain condoms		
Specify steps to using condoms correctly	Increased self-efficacy in using condoms		
Practise putting condoms over fingers			

How did they select the health goals?

- Through the review of quantitative data on STDs and pregnancy rates
- After consideration of the needs of the community

How did they select behaviours?

- Common knowledge about epidemiology
- The review of quantitative data, for example, survey data on sexual behaviour (note: all excluded some potentially important behaviours)
- After consideration of the needs of the community

How did they identify important risk and protective factors to target?

- Psychosocial theory, for example, theory of planned behaviour, social cognitive theory, theory of reasoned action
- Review of more than 500 studies of risk and protection (R&P) factors
- Interviews with professionals working with youth in the community
- Focus groups with young people

How did they identify or develop activities to change R&P factors?

- Psychosocial theory and educational theory (pedagogy)
- Review of activities in other curricula
- Development of new activities
- Pilot-tested activities

4. Designed activities consistent with community values and the resources available (staff time, staff skills, facility space and supplies)

5. Pilot-tested the program

Category 2: Characteristics describing the curriculum content

6. Focused on clear health goals – the prevention of STDs/HIV and/or pregnancy

- Talked about these health goals, including susceptibility and negative consequences
- Gave a clear message about these goals
- Identified behaviours leading to the health goal (see next characteristic)

7. Focused on specific behaviours leading to these health goals

- Specified behaviours
- Gave clear messages about these behaviours
- Addressed situations that might lead to them

What were the specific behaviours?
STD/HIV

- Abstinence and frequency of sex
- Number of partners (less commonly)
- Condom use

Pregnancy

- Abstinence and frequency of sex
- Contraceptive use

What was the clear message about behaviour?

- Emphasis on not having sex as the safest and best approach
- Encouraging condom/contraceptive use for those having sex
- Sometimes also emphasised other values, for example:

  1. Stick to your limits and remain in control (don't have sex if you don't want to, and use condoms if you do have sex)
  2. Be proud, be responsible, respect yourself

The clear messages were appropriate for age, sexual experience, gender and culture.

- Discussed specific situations that might lead to unwanted or unprotected sex and how to avoid them or get out of them
- Addressed multiple sexual psychosocial risk and protective factors affecting sexual behaviours

8. Addressed sexual psychological risk and protective factors that affect sexual behaviour

For abstinence

- Overall knowledge of sexual issues
- Knowledge of pregnancy, STDs and HIV condom/contraceptive use for those having sex and HIV risk
- Personal values about sex and abstinence
- Perception of peer norms about sex
- Self-efficacy to refuse sex
- Intention to abstain from sex or restrict sex or partners
- Communication with parents or other adults about sex, condoms or contraception

For condom and contraceptive use

- Knowledge of pregnancy, STDs and HIV
- Attitudes towards risky sexual behaviour and protection
- Attitudes towards condoms
- Perceived effectiveness of condoms to prevent STDs/HIV
- Perceptions of barriers to condom use
- Self-efficacy to obtain condoms

- Self-efficacy to use condoms
- Intention to use a condom
- Communication with parents or other adults about sex, condoms or contraception

9. Created a safe social environment in which youth can participate

- Created a safe social environment for youth to participate
- Established and enforced class rules
- Divided class by gender (occasionally)

10. Included multiple activities to change each of the targeted risk and protective factors

Included activities to increase basic knowledge about risks of teen sex and methods of avoiding sex or using protection

- Short lectures
- Class discussions
- Competitive games
- Simulations
- Statistics on prevalence
- Skits or videos
- Flip charts or pamphlets

Included activities to address risk (susceptibility and severity)

- Data on the incidence or prevalence of pregnancy or STDs/HIV (sometimes among youth) and their consequences
- Class discussions
- HIV+ speakers
- Videos, handouts, etc.
- Simulations, for example:
  1. STD handshake
  2. Monthly pregnancy risk
  3. Immediate and long-term effects on own lives

Included activities to change individual values about abstaining and perception of peer norms

- Clear message
- Advantages of abstinence
- Forced choice-value exercises
- Peer surveys/voting
- Peer modelling of responsible values
- Discussion of lines, role-plays

Included activities to change individual attitudes and peer norms about condoms

- Clear message
- Discussions of effectiveness
- Peer surveys/voting
- Discussions of barriers (where to get contraception, how to minimise hassle and the loss of enjoyment)
- Visits to drug stores or clinics
- Peer modelling of insisting on using condoms
- Discussion of lines, role-plays

Included activities to improve three skills

- To avoid unwanted sex and unprotected sex
- To insist on and use condom or contraception
- To use condoms correctly

To avoid unwanted/unprotected sex and to insist on using condoms or contraception

- Description of skills
- Modelling of skills
- Individual practice in skills through role-playing
  1. Everyone practises
  2. Repetition
  3. Increasing difficulty
  4. Increasing use of own words
- Feedback (for example, through a checklist)

How to use condoms properly

- Arrange in order the proper steps for using condoms
- Model and practise opening the package and putting condoms over fingers
- Verbally stating and following the important steps

Included instructionally effective activities to increase communication with parents or adults about sex (occasionally)

- Homework assignments
- Information sent home to parents
- Multiple assignments

11. Employed teaching methods that actively involved participants

- Instructionally sound, for example, using role-playing to improve skills
- Actively involved participants
- Personalising the information
- Small group discussions
- Brainstorming
- Games and contests
- Simulations of risk
- Role-playing
- Worksheets
- Other interactive experiential activities

12. Activities, instructional methods and behavioural messages appropriate to the youths' culture, developmental age, gender and sexual experience

- Be Proud; Be Responsible, focused on the needs of African-American youth
- SiHLE (Sistering, Informing, Healing, Living, and Empowering) focused on the needs of high risk women
- Many activities appropriately addressed abstinence versus condom use

13. Covered topics in a logical sequence

- Basic information about HIV, other STDs or pregnancy, including susceptibility and severity of HIV, other STDs and pregnancy
- Behaviours to reduce vulnerability
- Knowledge, values, attitudes (including perceived barriers) and social norms involving these behaviours
- Skills needed to perform these behaviours

Note: Curricula first increased the motivation to change behaviour, then provided knowledge, attitudes and skills to do so.

Category 3: Characteristics describing the implementation of the curriculum

14. Secured at least minimal support from appropriate authorities

- As these were research studies they required approval and support
- Provided sanction or support for educators

15. Selected educators with desired characteristics

Important selection criteria

- Could relate to youth
- Had experience with health education
- Were comfortable with the topic

Possibly **unimportant** *selection criteria*

- Age (adult versus peer)
- Matched gender or race

Training

- Virtually all studies involved trained educators
- One study showed the level of training had no impact

Supervision

- Monitoring
- Supervision
- Support (for example, discussed problems in small groups)

16. If needed, implemented activities to recruit and retain youth and overcome barriers to their involvement

- Publicised the programme
- Obtained parental consent
- Arranged for transportation
- Assured safety
- Implemented at convenient times
- Provided incentives to participate (for example, food)

17. Implemented virtually all activities with reasonable fidelity

- Most implemented activities that were planned
- Same setting or structure as designed

Conclusions about the Impact of Sex/HIV education programmes

- About two-thirds significantly improved behaviour
- Not all curricula were effective
- Most effective curricula incorporated the 17 characteristics
- Most curricula that included nearly all 17 characteristics were effective

The 17 characteristics of effective sex education

From *Emerging Answers 2007*: Characteristics of Effective Curriculum-Based Programs

THE PROCESS OF DEVELOPING THE CURRICULUM	THE CONTENTS OF THE CURRICULUM ITSELF	THE PROCESS OF IMPLEMENTING THE CURRICULUM
1. Involved multiple people with expertise in theory, research, and sex and STD/HIV education to develop the curriculum 2. Assessed relevant needs and assets of the target group 3. Used a logic model approach that specified the health goals, the types of behavior affecting those goals, the risk and protective factors affecting those types of behavior, and activities to change those risk and protective factors 4. Designed activities consistent with community values and available resources (e.g., staff time, staff skills, facility space and supplies) 5. Pilot-tested the program	CURRICULUM GOALS AND OBJECTIVES 6. Focused on clear health goals—the prevention of STD/HIV, pregnancy, or both 7. Focused narrowly on specific types of behavior leading to these health goals (e.g., abstaining from sex or using condoms or other contraceptives), gave clear messages about these types of behavior, and addressed situations that might lead to them and how to avoid them 8. Addressed sexual psychosocial risk and protective factors that affect sexual behavior (e.g., knowledge, perceived risks, values, attitudes, perceived norms, and self-efficacy) and changed them ACTIVITIES AND TEACHING METHODOLOGIES 9. Created a safe social environment for young people to participate 10. Included multiple activities to change each of the targeted risk and protective factors 11. Employed instructionally sound teaching methods that actively involved participants, that helped them personalize the information, and that were designed to change the targeted risk and protective factors 12. Employed activities, instructional methods, and behavioral messages that were appropriate to the teens' culture, developmental age, and sexual experience 13. Covered topics in a logical sequence	14. Secured at least minimal support from appropriate authorities, such as departments of health, school districts, or community organizations 15. Selected educators with desired characteristics (whenever possible), trained them, and provided monitoring, supervision, and support 16. If needed, implemented activities to recruit and retain teens and overcome barriers to their involvement (e.g., publicized the program, offered food or obtained consent) 17. Implemented virtually all activities with reasonable fidelity

Conclusion and next steps for sex and relationships education

SEF's 21st Birthday Conference on Thursday 23 October 2008 was an historic day that will stay in the memories of the delegates and speakers for many years. On this day, not only did the Minister for Schools and Learners, Rt Hon Jim Knight, announce that PSHE will become a statutory part of the curriculum, but the government also published a set of measures to improve SRE. These measures were based on recommendations made following a review of SRE in schools undertaken by an External Steering Group to which SEF contributed.

The following outlines the next steps for SRE, based on the government's response to the SRE Review. The Sex Education Forum welcomes these measures and looks forward to supporting the government to ensure that they are undertaken. We hope to report a significant improvement in sex and relationships education by SEF's 25th Birthday in 2012.

Recommendations to improve SRE. What will happen next?

PSHE

A review into how best to make PSHE statutory will be conducted and will report by April 2009. Following this, there will be a full public consultation on the statutory programmes of study. Schools will then have a year to prepare, making it likely that statutory PSHE will be implemented in September 2011.

SRE

The Review Group identified six specific, plus some non-specific, areas where action needs to be taken.

1. Improving the skills and confidence of those who deliver PSHE

- Provision of materials to support INSET on duty to promote well-being and, more specifically, to improve the quality of SRE with a particular focus on raising awareness of the whole school workforce

- Funding for existing CPD-PSHE programmes committed to 2010–11; funding to be made available for an increase in the number of teachers participating annually (currently between 1,500 and 2,000); evidence of impact of CPD programme on improving quality of PSHE delivery to be gathered

- Shorter, more knowledge-based, courses on SRE to be promoted

- For Initial Teacher Training (ITT), commitment from the TDA to pilot places to specialise as PSHE teachers; questions to be added to Newly Qualified Teacher surveys to assess ITT preparation for PSHE teaching and promoting well-being; recognition of the need to promote a PSHE career path to both potential teachers and schools

- New briefing for governors to raise awareness of new well-being duty and its relationship to SRE

2. Encouraging the use of external contributors to support schools' delivery of SRE

- Local PSHE Healthy School Leads to be encouraged to develop directories of organisations that can support SRE in schools, in accordance with SEF's Guidance (Forum Factsheet 8) on external contributors to PSHE

- New guidance will encourage schools to adopt a whole school approach to PSHE, in which PSHE teachers are supported by external contributors, who in turn should be trained and integrated into the programme

3. The case for further guidance and support for schools on SRE

The existing SRE Guidance (2000) will be updated by a group including key stakeholders, taking more account of what young people want to be included and at what key stage; it will be inclusive and relevant to all young people, and focus more on relationships. The draft Guidance will be consulted on widely. It will cover the following.

- Provide examples of different approaches to SRE delivery, including those taken by faith schools

- Set out the topics to be covered and a common core of information and skills for all young people

- Allow schools to determine their own approach to the teaching of sensitive issues in line with the school's ethos and views of the parents

The Review Group identified the following key principles necessary to underpin future guidance to improve the delivery of SRE.

- A stronger focus in SRE on relationships and the skills and values that young people need

- SRE should be set within a clear and explicit values framework of mutual respect, rights and responsibilities, gender equality and acceptance of diversity

- SRE should be inclusive and meet the needs of all young people, including recognition of issues such as sexuality, disability, ethnicity and faith

- SRE needs to complement the wider provision of information, advice and support to young people on sex and relationships

- Schools need to do more to inform parents about what SRE they are delivering in each key stage

- Schools should work in partnership with external professionals working in health and wider children's services

- SRE should not be taught in isolation and links need to be made with other parts of the PSHE curriculum

4. Involving young people in the design of SRE programmes

- DCSF (Department for Children, Schools and Families) will promote SEF's SRE Pupil Audit Toolkit for consulting with young people, building it more formally into the National Healthy Schools Programme and the National CPD-PSHE Programme

- A new question to be added to the 'TellUs' survey, 'Did SRE in school meet your needs?'

- A question about young people's perceptions of SRE has been proposed in Ofsted well-being indicators (currently out for consultation)

- Assessment in PSHE should be brought in line with practice in other curriculum subjects

5. Maximising the impact of wider government programmes on improving SRE delivery

- New guidance on PSHE was published by the National Healthy Schools Programme in November 2008, which illustrates what evidence schools should supply to demonstrate that they are meeting PSHE criteria, and a Revised Quality Assurance Guidance is due to be issued early in 2009, to ensure a more rigorous assessment that schools meet the standards for SRE

- New supplementary SEAL (Social and Emotional Aspects of Learning) materials on sexual relationships to be developed for schools

- DCSF to produce briefing for local authorities and PCTs to encourage them to take a more strategic role in improving the quality of SRE in schools and as a means of demonstrating the attainment of national indicators, including a reduction in under-18 conceptions and Chlamydia prevalence.

6. Improving leadership on SRE

- NCSL (National College for School Leadership) to consider how to promote SRE with school leaders, over and above measures to make PSHE statutory

7. Other issues

- DCSF 'SRE and Parents' leaflet to be revised to include a summary of the new guidance on what should be taught at each key stage and to emphasise the partnership with parents

- SRE for post-16 learners is not fully considered within timescale of this review, however proposals for SRE through further education (FE) and work-based learning will be developed, building on SEF's work on developing health advice services in FE; in addition, joint DCSF, DH and DIUS (*Department for Innovation, Universities and Skills*) proposals for a 'Healthy College' framework are currently in development

- Further research and evaluation of SRE will be considered

- Re-branding SRE to be considered

For further information see the full reports, *Review of Sex and Relationship Education (SRE) in Schools – A Report by the External Steering Group* and *Government Response to the Report by the Sex and Relationships Education (SRE) Review Steering Group* (Ref: DCSF-00860-2008) which can be found at: www.teachernet.gov.uk/publications

Programme

Celebrating Sex and Relationships Education:
Past, Present and Future
Sex Education Forum 21st Birthday Conference

Scope and aims

SEF believes that all children and young people have the right to good quality SRE. Over the last 21 years, we have been working with our diverse membership to make this right become a reality.

This is an exciting time for SRE. Schools now have a statutory duty to ensure the well-being of their pupils and SRE makes a vital contribution to this. Furthermore, the government has recently undertaken a review of SRE with support from SEF. As a result, recommendations will be made to improve the status and delivery of SRE within PSHE.

With high levels of STIs, pregnancy and ignorance on sex and relationships matters amongst young people in England, there continues to be a need to raise the profile of SRE. We also need to understand and showcase best practice and to support professionals who deliver this subject, both in schools and other settings.

This conference offers a unique opportunity to move the agenda forward and for professionals to network with others in the field and take away learning about SRE.

Delegates at this one-day national conference will:

- look at SRE from a variety of perspectives, including key achievements over the past 21 years, the current policy context and the future
- discuss new ideas and good practice, and determine what constitutes effective SRE

Who should attend?

All professionals involved in the promotion, design and/or delivery of SRE either in or out of school settings, including:

- SRE teachers
- PSHE teachers
- School nurses
- SRE educators from other settings such as the voluntary, youth or community sector
- PSHE coordinators and leads
- Teenage Pregnancy coordinators
- Healthy Schools coordinators

Programme

Sex Education Forum: 21st Birthday Conference

Thursday 23 October 2008, Central Hall, Westminster

9.30   **Registration and refreshments**

10.00   **Welcome and introduction**
Jane Lees, Chair, Sex Education Forum

10.10   **How did we get here? 21 years of sex and relationships education**
Anna Martinez, Coordinator, Sex Education Forum

10.25   **What have we learnt? What works, what doesn't and ways forward: international evidence**
Douglas Kirby, Senior Research Scientist, ETR Associates

10.45   **What do we want? The launch of the Young People's Charter for SRE**
Adam Lonsdale, Alex Helliwell and Ella Durant

11.00   **What is the future for SRE? The government's response to the Review of SRE in schools**
Rt Hon Jim Knight MP, Minister for Schools and Learners

11.30   **Refreshments**

12.00   **First choice of workshops**

Workshop 1: Social norms and SRE – sharing examples from schools in Bedfordshire of the normative approach
Andi Whitwham, Drug, Alcohol and Sex and Relationships consultant

Workshop 2: Rude, crude and socially unacceptable. Young people and pornography
Mark Limmer, Deputy Regional Teenage Pregnancy Coordinator

Workshop 3: Parents – building bridges between parents and schools
David Kesterton, project manager, Speakeasy, fpa

Workshop 4: Involving young people – using the 'Are You Getting It Right?' Pupil Audit Toolkit to consult young people on SRE
Lesley de Meza, co-author of the Toolkit, PSHE education consultant, trainer and writer

Workshop 5: Faith and Values – exploring SRE in a multi-faith society looking at local case studies
Sarah Thistle, Change for Children manager, VTE&S
Hansa Patel-Kanwal, independent consultant and life member of SEF

Workshop 6: 'Scored project' – working creatively, using football, to engage with vulnerable young people in SRE
Karina Bowkett, Winner of the Pamela Sheridan Award 2008

Workshop 7: What works? 17 characteristics of effective sex education
Douglas Kirby, Senior Research Scientist, ETR Associates

13.15 Lunch

14.15 Second choice of workshops

15.30 Close of conference

15.45 Birthday drinks reception
Welcome address by Anne Weyman, founder of SEF

Speaker biographies

Jane Lees
Chair, Sex Education Forum
Jane began her career teaching SRE. Presently, as an fpa trainer and CPD-PSHE Lead, Jane trains other teachers to teach SRE with confidence.

Jane has advised schools as well as local and central government about the implementation of SRE and has written national frameworks and guidance. She has worked with successive education departments and the QCA. Jane has made a significant contribution to the inclusion of PSHE in the national curriculum through leading the national PSHE advisory group.

Jane has also worked, through Unicef, on the national life skills curricula in Moldova, Jordan, Azerbaijan and Macedonia. Previous roles include ILEA Inspector for Health Education and Personal Development and as a local authority senior officer. Prior to taking up her new role as Chair of SEF, Jane chaired NSCoPSE – the National PSE Association for advisors, inspectors and consultants – for eight years and represented it on SEF for longer.

Anna Martinez
Coordinator, Sex Education Forum
Anna Martinez has been the Coordinator of SEF since 2003. SEF, a unique collaboration of 50 organisations and a leading authority on SRE, works to ensure that all children and young people receive their right to good quality SRE. In 2008 Anna represented SEF on the External Steering Group for the review of SRE in schools. She is also a member of the NICE Programme Development Group for PSHE guidance.

Anna has an MSc in Health Promotion Sciences from the London School of Hygiene and Tropical Medicine, and is a qualified sexual health trainer. Before joining SEF Anna worked for a local Teenage Pregnancy team specialising in professional training in SRE. Anna has also worked for UNAIDS on HIV prevention.

Anna Martinez has co-authored a variety of SRE resources: *Effective Learning Methods: Approaches to Teaching about Sex and Relationships within PSHE and Citizenship; Laying the Foundations. Sex and Relationships Education in Primary Schools*; and *'Are You Getting It Right?' A Toolkit for Consulting Young People on Sex and Relationships Education.*

Douglas Kirby
Senior Research Scientist, ETR Associates
Douglas Kirby, PhD, is a Senior Research Scientist at ETR Associates. For about 30 years, he has directed state-wide or nation-wide studies of adolescent sexual behaviour, abstinence-only programmes, sex and STD/HIV education programmes, school-based clinics, school condom-availability programmes and youth development programmes. He co-authored research on the *Reducing the Risk, Safer Choices* and *Draw the Line* curricula, all of which significantly reduced unprotected sex, either by delaying sex, reducing the number of partners, increasing condom use or by increasing contraceptive use. He has summarised the effects of programmes designed to reduce adolescent sexual risk and has published these summaries in such widely recognised volumes as *Emerging Answers 2007*. In these reviews, he has identified important common characteristics of effective sex education and STD/HIV education programmes.

Adam Lonsdale
Adam joined his local youth council in 2007 and quickly became a member of the Sexual Health Group. The Sexual Health Group has made strong progress in tackling homophobic posters and has organised a world AIDS day gig. Adam also took on the UK Youth Parliament opportunity and became one of two representatives for East Riding of Yorkshire.

Sexual health is Adam's highest priority issue, and he advocates passionately for SRE to be tackled in schools. Adam does all he can to help and enjoys the work he does. In the future Adam would like to progress further in the fields of politics or medicine. Adam has spoken on the radio, and to multiple councillors in the past, and has also delivered a sex education lesson to a group of 270 Year 9s.

Alex Helliwell
Alex Helliwell believes strongly that young people's voices need to be heard and has spoken at national conferences about this topic. He is also involved in assisting UNICEF to promote their campaign to prevent HIV in the UK and abroad. Currently he is reading Politics, Sociology and Psychology at St Catharine's College, Cambridge.

Esther Olayiwola
Esther is a student at Seven Kings High School and studying Biology, Chemistry, English Literature and Mathematics. Esther has been involved with youth politics for two years, having been a member of Newham Youth Parliament and now Newham Youth Council.

SRE has been one of the major issues that the Youth Parliament has worked on, introducing Sexual Health Information News Exchange (SHINE) workshops to the local community and starting up a lifestyle brand called LoveLife.

Ella Durant

Ella is 17 years old and is a dedicated, committed, outgoing young person who has helped to rewrite the national SRE Charter. Ella is currently doing A levels in Politics, Art and Drama and AS History and Psychology.

Next year Ella plans to study a Drama and Politics combined degree at university or take a gap year out as a youth worker. She would like to pursue a career involving youth politics or drama.

Ella is a Deputy Member of the Youth Parliament for South Somerset and has been involved for four years. She has worked passionately on many elements of the manifesto campaigns, attended many events and been a part of many relevant groups. Ella's biggest commitment has been to the SRE campaign. Some of the things Ella has done whilst campaigning include: the SRE element of a local campaign film, giving a speech on SRE at the local MYP results evening, speaking about SRE in a meeting with local counsellors, reviewing SRE resources, mystery shopping at an SRE clinic, shadowing an SRE in schools deliverer leader for takeover day, attending an 'educating primary schools on how to deliver SRE' conference training day and speaking with different schools voicing young people's opinions.

Rt Hon Jim Knight MP
Minister of State for Schools and Learners

Jim Knight's principal policy areas include raising school standards including public examinations and national tests, the national curriculum, 14–19 education and diplomas, school funding and capital, including Building Schools for the Future, and school workforce issues.

Jim Knight was first appointed Minister of State to the then Department for Education and Skills in May 2006. Previously Minister for Rural Affairs, Landscape and Biodiversity since the 2005 general election, Jim Knight was elected MP for Dorset South in June 2001.

He served as Parliamentary Private Secretary to Rosie Winterton at the Department of Health between 2003 and 2004, before going on to serve as PPS to the Department of Health's ministerial team.

Jim Knight, 41, was educated at Cambridge. Before entering parliament, he managed a publishing company, based in the West Country, for 10 years. Prior to that, he managed arts venues and worked for a small-scale travelling theatre company. He is married with two children.

Andi Whitwham
Drug, Alcohol and Sex and Relationships consultant
Andi Whitwham is currently the Bedfordshire Drug, Alcohol and Sex and Relationships consultant for upper and special schools. She first worked in Derbyshire in a challenging secondary school for two years and then in Bedfordshire for twenty-four years, first as a teacher in a middle school and then in her present post. She has had particular success in encouraging upper schools to deliver PSHE with specialist teams of teachers. She is also responsible for supporting schools in achieving National Healthy School Status as part of the Bedfordshire Healthy Schools Team and is also involved in the delivery of the National CPD-PSHE Programme to teachers and school nurses. Her latest role is as manager of Student Consultants for Children and Young people, promoting student voice initiatives both locally and nationally. Andi also works closely with the police, and young people's drug, alcohol and sexual health services to promote their work in schools.

As part of her consultancy work she is responsible for reviewing policies and programmes for drugs and SRE, developing and delivering training programmes specific to needs and for working with schools in challenging circumstances. Andi has just completed the first year of the social norms pilot in five upper schools across the county. She is further developing the social norms project into its second year to include more schools and has extended the work to involve schools from outside Bedfordshire. This year there are two special projects, which will involve intensive work in schools using various agencies and different subject departments within the schools to consolidate and extend the work around social norms education.

Mark Limmer
Deputy Regional Teenage Pregnancy Coordinator
Mark Limmer is currently the Deputy Regional Teenage Pregnancy Coordinator for the north-west of England and for the last 20 years has worked in the field of young people's sexual health as a youth and community worker, health advisor, psychotherapist, trainer and strategist.

Mark has a particular interest in working with and researching young men, particularly young men whose sexual attitudes and behaviours are seen as problematic. Mark has an MA in Health Research from the University of Lancashire and is currently writing up his doctoral research, which focuses on the impact of masculinity and exclusion on sexual risk-taking among young men. Mark's other research interests include exploring the links between alcohol use and sexual health in young people and the development of effective policy and practice to improve the emotional and physical sexual health of excluded and vulnerable young men and women.

David Kesterton
Project manager, Speakeasy, fpa

David has been project manager for Speakeasy at fpa since January 2002. In addition to overseeing the development of the programme across the UK, he has piloted the work in a number of European countries. In 2008 David sat on the ministerial review of SRE representing the perspective of parents.

Prior to fpa David worked in the voluntary sector as a manager in an HIV support service in London and a 'One Stop Shop' information and advice service for 13–25 year olds in Bedfordshire. Originally ordained in the Church of England where he worked in the dioceses of Litchfield and St Albans, David has considerable experience of group-based learning programmes for adults and young people in community settings and of partnership working at local and strategic levels. A parent and 'step parent', David lives in Bedfordshire with his partner and children aged between 11 and 17. In 2008 he was invited to become a fellow of the Royal Society of Arts, Manufacturing and Design.

Lesley de Meza
Independent practitioner, trainer and writer

Lesley Michele de Meza is a leading practitioner, trainer and writer known internationally for her PSHE education work. She was a member of the Interim Council of the PSHE Association and worked as part of a QCA project team on Personal and Social Development curriculum materials and case studies.

Lesley works with many organisations including: DAATs, DCSF, DoH, HIT (Liverpool), Home Office, IYSS, local authorities, the Metropolitan Police, NICE, PCTs, QCA, schools, TPU and universities.

In November 2008 Lesley was appointed as an 'Education Practitioner' member of the Public Health Interventions Advisory Committee (PHIAC), which is part of the National Institute for Health & Clinical Excellence (NICE). She is also an associate trainer for NCB and Brook. Her 2008 publications include: *Are You Getting it Right? A Toolkit for Consulting Young People on SRE*, written with Anna Martinez; *Risk Taking* written with Paul Law; *Drugs Education for KS2*, BBC Whiteboard Active series; and *PSHE Education 1*, co-written with Stephen de Silva.

Sarah Thistle
Change for Children Manager, VTE&S

Sarah Thistle is Change for Children manager in the London Borough of Waltham Forest, where she oversees the local healthy schools programme (including SRE), advisory support for community cohesion and citizenship, anti bullying work and the Learning Mentor Programme. She has previously worked in primary and special schools and set up work-based family learning projects at Ford Motor Company. Sarah also spent 18 months as Senior Development Officer at the Sex Education Forum, where she contributed to the development of the DfES Teachernet PSHE website and led on the Secondary Schools and Services and Primary School projects.

Hansa Patel-Kanwal OBE
Independent Consultant
Hansa Patel Kanwal OBE is an Independent Consultant working on organisational development and sexual health issues, with particular expertise in the development and delivery of culturally and linguistically appropriate service provision for a range of black and minority ethnic communities.

Hansa has co-authored *Lets Talk about Sex and Relationships: A Policy and Practice Framework for Working with Children and Young People in Public Care, Let's Make it Happen: Training on Sex, Relationships, Pregnancy and Parenthood for Those Working with Looked After Children and Young People* and has compiled a 'Positive Woman's Survival Kit' for HIV-positive women.

Hansa has also produced *Guidelines for Service Providers on Sexual Health work and Hindu Communities* and *Guidance for Developing Contraception and Sexual Health Advice Services to Reach Black and Minority Ethnic Young People.*

Hansa is a member of the Independent Advisory Group on Teenage Pregnancy, advising government on the implementation of the National Teenage Pregnancy Strategy.

Karina Bowkett
The Young People's Health Project, Birmingham
Karina graduated from Liverpool University with a BSc (Hons) Health and Physical Recreation in 2003. After working in Australia and travelling for almost a year Karina then settled back in Birmingham. Karina is a new recruit to Birmingham Youth Service and has been working for the Young People's Health Project for just 15 months. Prior to this her background was in the health service and her previous job was with Birmingham and Solihull Mental Health Foundation Trust as Social Inclusion Coordinator and also with Solihull MBC Youth Service. Karina's role as an holistic health project worker has meant she has had the flexibility to respond to the local health needs of young people and develop creative projects to deliver key health messages to young people in the way they want. She believes that effective SRE is a result of meaningful consultation with young people. Karina has recently started the CPD-PSHE certificate.

Michelle Thompson
The Young People's Health Project, Birmingham
Michelle Thompson joined the Young People's Health Project three years ago as a sexual health project worker. During this time she has had the opportunity to be part of various practical programmes, enabling her to engage with a diverse group of young people around the issues of sexual health and help them to make informed choices around sex and relationships. Michelle has a young daughter herself and as a young parent believes in the importance of delivering SRE that captures young people where they are at, in order to support them in making informed choices concerning sex and relationships. Alongside SRE delivery, earlier this year she completed her Youth Work Diploma. Over the next year she will be completing her BPhil degree in Youth Work studies. This is Michelle's first conference workshop and she is really excited about being here today.

Chris McCabe
The Young People's Health Project, Birmingham
Chris McCabe graduated with a BA (Hons) in Combined Health Studies in 1997, with a particular interest in health promotion and working with young people.

Chris has worked with the Young People's Health Project, which is part of the Birmingham Youth Service, Children, Young People and Families Directorate, for eight years as their full time sexual health project worker. Over this time Chris has worked with many young people in a variety of settings and on a number of sexual health projects. Many of these young people have been vulnerable, with multiple needs, and have included young people from Youth Inclusion, alternative learning programmes, those excluded from school and NEET young people.

She worked extensively on establishing Young People's Sexual Health drop-ins in her local area in the east of Birmingham and also on the development of an SRE programme for use in local secondary schools. Chris has developed and delivered training and contributed to sexual health policies within the local area for the Youth Service in Birmingham, and also led on the development of health resources for use with young people around a number of health issues.

More recently she has been involved in the consultation and development of targeted prevention work and the shaping of local teenage pregnancy implementation plans.

Chris has also undertaken a huge amount of work with young parents, establishing in her early days the first young parents' support group in Birmingham provided by the statutory services with a local health visitor. She has also run targeted alternative learning programmes for young parents and worked on projects tackling the stigma and isolation faced by young parents as well as resource development.

Delegate list

Sex Education Forum, 21st Birthday Celebration

Thursday 23rd October 2008, Central Hall, Westminster

To respect the privacy of delegates, names have been removed. Delegates are listed by job title or SEF membership

Advisor for PSHE and Citizenship, London Borough of Sutton
Advisor for PSHE and Citizenship, Wiltshire County Council
Advisor for PSHE and Healthy Schools, East Sussex County Council
Assistant Head, Aylesbury Vale Secondary Support Centre
Assistant Head, James Brindley School
Biology/PSHE Teacher, Bedales School
Campaign Coordinator, Respect Yourself, Warwickshire County Council
Centre Manager, Brook Advisory Service
CEO, Health Behaviour Group
Chair of TPIAG
Chair of Trustees, Health Behaviour Group
Children's Centre Manager, Cambridgeshire County Council
Consultant PSHE and Healthy Schools, East Sussex County Council (x4)
Curriculum Advisor PSHE, Harrow Council
Development and Training Manager, TACADE
Development Officer, Wigan MBC
Director of Health, Oasis Trust
Drug Education Trainer, Wigan MBC
Drug Education/PSHE Consultant, Bristol City Council
Education Development Officer, Healthy Schools, North East Lincolnshire Council
Executive Director, British Medical Association
Freelance Education Consultant
Head of PSHCE, Wye Valley School
Head of PSHE and Citizenship, Richard's Lodge High School
Head of PSHE/Head of Year 8, Mount School
Health Improvement Officer, Royal Borough Kensington and Chelsea
Health Improvement Practitioner, South Tyneside PCT
Health Improvement Specialist (Young People's Sexual Health), Westminster PCT
Health Improvement Specialist, County Durham and Darlington PCT
Health Improvement Specialist, Leeds PCT
Healthy Schools Advisor, Northamptonshire PCT
Healthy Schools Consultant, Coventry City Council

Healthy Schools Consultant, Hertfordshire County Council
Healthy Schools Consultant, Teenage Pregnancy, Rotherham Metropolitan Borough
    Council
Healthy Schools Coordinator, Coventry City Council
Healthy Schools Coordinator, Cumbria Children's Services
Healthy Schools Coordinator, East Riding of Yorkshire Council
Healthy Schools Coordinator, Government Office North West
Healthy Schools Link Advisor, London Borough of Croydon Council
Healthy Schools Programme Manager, Leicestershire County Council
Healthy Schools Programme Manager, South West Essex PCT
Independent Consultant
Independent Consultant, JBR Associates
Independent Consultant, Strategic Choice Limited
Independent Education Consultant, The Christopher Winter Project
Instructor, Sharnbrook Upper School and Community College
Interim Head of Public Affairs, UNICEF
Lambeth Schools SRE Coordinator, Lambeth PCT
Learning Consultant, London Borough of Enfield Council
Lecturer in Personal and Social Education, University of Cambridge School of
    Education
Life Member, Sex Education Forum
London Borough of Newham (Education Department)
National Director, Life Education Centres
National School Support Officer, Church of England
Outreach Nurse, Brook
Parent (x1)
Pastoral Carer, William Read Primary School
Personal Development Consultant, Stoke on Trent City Council
PhD Student, University of Manchester
Policy Advisor, House of Commons
Policy and Development Manager, Brook
Policy Development Officer, YMCA
Policy Manager, Parentline Plus
Practice Development Director, fpa
Project Worker, Education for Choice
PSHCE Consultant, Bedfordshire County Council
PSHCE Coordinator, William Read Primary School
PSHE Advisor and Head of Health Through Education, London Borough of Tower
    Hamlets
PSHE Consultant, Blackpool Council
PSHE Consultant, Education Leeds
PSHE Consultant, Stoke on Trent City Council
PSHE Coordinator, Davenant Foundation School
PSHE Coordinator, East Riding of Yorkshire Council
PSHE Coordinator, Peterborough City Council
PSHE/Citizenship Coordinator, Wakefield Healthy Schools
Public Health Strategist, Tower Hamlets PCT

Pupil Well-being, Health and Safety Unit, Department for Children, Schools and Families
Regional Sex Education Coordinator, Telford and Wrekin Council
Research Consultant, Me-and-Us
Research Officer, Teens and Toddlers
Retired Lecturer
School Improvement Officer – PSHE/Citizenship, London Borough of Enfield Council
School Nurse, Birmingham East and North PCT (x3)
School Nurse, Bolton Metropolitan Borough Council
School Nurse, Bromley PCT
School Nurse, West Sussex PCT
School Support Worker – HIV, Lambeth PCT
Senior Advisor, PSHE Association
Senior Consultant – Healthy Schools, Education Leeds
Senior Lecturer, Middlesex University
Senior Manager/Oasis Educator, 2XL Youth Projects
Senior Practitioner, Barnardos
Senior School Nurse, West Sussex PCT
Sex and Relationships Education Advisor, Cornwall and Isles of Scilly PCT
Sex and Relationships Education Advisor, Somerset County Council
Sex and Relationships Education Consultant, Buckinghamshire County Council
Sexual Health Nurse, Harrow Council
Sexual Health Nurse Advisor, West Sussex PCT
Sexual Health Outreach, Brook
Sexual Health Promotion/Education Nurse, Isle of Wight NHS PCT
Sexual Health Team Lead, Isle of Wight NHS PCT
Somerset County Council
Speakeasy Development Worker, Speakeasy
Speakeasy Learning Mentor, Speakeasy
Specialist Nurse for Young People, Lambeth PCT
Specialist Sexual Health Nurse, Croydon PCT
SRE Advisor, Luton Borough Council
SRE Advisor, Swindon Borough Council
SRE Advisor, Warrington Borough Council
SRE and Drugs Advisor, VTPLC
SRE and Drugs Consultant, Bedfordshire County Council
SRE Consultant, Barnsley Metropolitan Borough Council
SRE Consultant, Gloucestershire County Council
SRE Development Officer, Bolton Metropolitan Borough Council
SRE Development Worker, Tower Hamlets PCT
SRE Trainer, The Christopher Winter Project
SRE Training and Development Specialist, Croydon PCT
SRE Training Coordinator, Isle of Wight County Council
Staff/School Nurse, Bromley PCT
Strategy Manager/ Chair of Advisory Council, London Borough of Camden
Sutton Teenage Pregnancy Coordinator, Sutton and Merton PCT
Teacher Advisor for Healthy Schools, Portsmouth City Council

Teacher Advisor for PSHE/Healthy Schools, Worcestershire County Council
Teacher Advisor for SRE, North East Lincolnshire Council
Teaching and Learning Advisor, South Gloucestershire Council
Team Leader, Department for Children, Schools and Families
Teenage Pregnancy Coordinator, Croydon PCT
Teenage Pregnancy Coordinator, East Riding of Yorkshire Council
Teenage Pregnancy Coordinator, East Sussex County Council
Teenage Pregnancy Coordinator, Somerset County Council
Teenage Pregnancy Coordinator, Westminster City Council
Teenage Pregnancy Lead, Birmingham East and North PCT
Teenage Pregnancy Strategy Coordinator, North Yorkshire County Council
Teenage Pregnancy Training Coordinator, Blackpool Council
Teenage Pregnancy Youth Representative, Wiltshire Assembly of Youth
Training and Development Manager, Health Behaviour Group
Training Manager, Deafax
TYS Substance Misuse and Sexual Health Worker, Slough Borough Council
UK Youth Parliament
Young Gay Men's Development Officer, Terrence Higgins Trust
Youth Support Drug Misuse and Sexual Health, Slough Borough Council
Youth Worker, Brook

Bibliography

How did we get here? 21 years of sex and relationships education (SRE)

Blake, S. and Frances, G. (2001) *Just Say No to Abstinence Education: Lessons Learnt from a Sex Education Study Tour to the United States*. London: National Children's Bureau.

Bosche, S. (1983) *Jenny Lives with Eric and Martin*. London: Gay Men's Press.

Clyde, C. (2001) *Understanding Schools and Schooling*. London: Routledge

Department for Education and Employment (1993) *Education Act 1993: Sex Education in Schools (Circular 5/94)*. London: DfEE.

Department for Education and Employment (1999) *National Healthy School Standard: Guidance*. London: DfEE.

Department for Education and Employment (2000) *Sex and Relationship Education Guidance (0116/2000)*. London: DfEE.

Education (No. 2) Act 1986. London: HMSO.
http://www.opsi.gov.uk/acts/acts1986/pdf/ukpga_19860061_en.pdf

Education Act 1993. London: HMSO.
http://www.opsi.gov.uk/acts/acts1993/pdf/ukpga_19930035_en.pdf

Education Act 1996. London: HMSO.
http://www.opsi.gov.uk/acts/acts1996/Ukpga_19960056_en_1

Education and Inspections Act 2006. London: Stationery Office.
http://www.opsi.gov.uk/acts/acts2006/pdf/ukpga_20060040_en.pdf

'Framework for personal, social and health education at key stages 3 & 4', in Qualifications and Curricu lum Authority (1999) *The National Curriculum: Handbook for Secondary Teachers in England, Key Stages 3 and 4*. London: DfEE/QCA.

Johnson, A.M. and others (1994) *Sexual Attitudes and Lifestyles*. Oxford: Blackwell Scientific Publications.

Local Government Act 1988. London: HMSO.
http://www.opsi.gov.uk/acts/acts1988/pdf/ukpga_19880009_en.pdf

Local Government Act 2003. London: Stationery Office.

http://www.opsi.gov.uk/acts/acts2003/pdf/ukpga_20030026_en.pdf

Martinez, A. (2006) *Beyond Biology*. London: National Children's Bureau.
http://www.ncb.org.uk/dotpdf/open_access_2/beyond_biology_p9.pdf

Qualifications and Curriculum Authority (2007) *Personal Well-being: Non-statutory Programmes of Study for Key Stage 3 and Key Stage 4*. London: QCA.
http://curriculum.qca.org.uk/key-stages-3-and-4/subjects/pshe/index.aspx

Sex Education Forum (2000) *Young People's Charter for Good Sex and Relationships Education*. London: SEF.

Sexual Offences (Amendment) Act 2000. London: Stationery Office.

Sexual Offences Act 2003. London: Stationery Office.
http://www.opsi.gov.uk/acts/acts2003/pdf/ukpga_20030042_en.pdf

Social Exclusion Unit (1999) *Teenage Pregnancy (Cm 4342)*. London: Stationery Office.

Thomson, R. (ed.) (1993) *Religion, Ethnicity and Sex Education: Exploring the Issues*. London: National Children's Bureau on behalf of the Sex Education Forum.

Thomson, R. and Scott, L. (1992) *An Enquiry into Sex Education: Report of a Survey into Local Education Authority Support and Monitoring of School Sex Education*. London: National Children's Bureau on behalf of the Sex Education Forum.

UK Youth Parliament (2007) *SRE: Are You Getting It?* London: UK Youth Parliament.
http://www.ukyouthparliament.org.uk/campaigns/sre/AreYouGettingIt.pdf

What have we learnt? What works, what doesn't and ways forward: international evidence

Kirby, D. (2007) *Emerging Answers 2007: Research Findings on Programs to Reduce Teen Pregnancy and Sexually Transmitted Diseases*. Washington, DC: National Campaign to Prevent Teen and Unplanned Pregnancy.

Kirby, D. (2008) 'The impact of abstinence and comprehensive sex and STD/HIV education programs on adolescent sexual behavior', *Sexuality Research and Social Policy*, 5, 3, 18–27.

Kirby, D., Laris, B.A. and Rolleri, L. (2007) 'The impact of sex and HIV education programs in schools and communities on sexual behaviors among adolescents and young adults', *Journal of Adolescent Health*, 40, 3, 206–217.

Kirby, D., Rolleri, L. and Wilson, M.M. (2007) *Tool to Assess the Characteristics of Effective Sex and STD/HIV education programs (TAC)*. Washington DC: Healthy Teen Network.

What do we want to see in the future? The launch of the Young People's Charter for SRE

HM Treasury (2003) *Every Child Matters (Cm 5860)*. London: Stationery Office.

Sex Education Forum (2008) *We Want More! What Young People Want from Sex and Relationships Education. Charter for Change*. London: National Children's Bureau.

United Nations (1989) *The Convention on the Rights of the Child*. Adopted by the General Assembly of the United Nations on 20 November 1989. Geneva: Defence for Children International and the United Nations Children's Fund.

What is the future for SRE? The government's response to the SRE Review

Department for Children, Schools and Families (2008) *Government Response to the Report by the Sex and Relationships Education (SRE) Review Steering Group*. London: DCSF. http://www.teachernet.gov.uk/_doc/13030/7924-DCSF-Sex%20and%20Relationships%20A4.pdf

Dickens, C. (2003) *A Tale of Two Cities*. London: Penguin.

New York Times Magazine 'A Teenage Bill of Rights', in Savage, J. (2007) *Teenage: The Creation of Youth 1875–1945*. London: Chatto & Windus. p455.

Rousseau, J.J. 'Rousseau's second birth of adolescence. *Emile*', in Savage, J. (2007) *Teenage: The Creation of Youth 1875–1945*. London: Chatto & Windus. p13.

SRE Review Steering Group (2008) *Review of Sex and Relationship Education (SRE) in Schools: A Report by the External Steering Group.* London: DCSF. http://www.teachernet.gov.uk/_doc/13030/SRE%20final.pdf

Workshops

Workshop 1: Social norms and SRE – sharing examples from schools in Bedfordshire of the normative approach

Perkins, H.W. (2003) *The Social Norms Approach to Preventing School and College Age Substance Abuse.* San Francisco: Jossey-Bass.

de Silva, S. and Blake, S. (2006) *Positive Guidance on Aspects of Personal, Social and Health Education.* London: National Children's Bureau.

Workshop 2: Rude, crude and socially unacceptable. Young people and pornography

Carroll, J. and others (2008) 'Generation XXX: pornography acceptance and use among emerging adults', *Journal of Adolescent Research,* 23, 6, 6–30.

Epstein, D. and Johnson, R. (1998) *Schooling Sexualities.* Buckingham: Oxford University Press.

Fisher, W. and Barak, A. (2001) 'Internet pornography: a social psychological perspective on Internet sexuality', *Journal of Sex Research,* 38, 4, 312–323.

Haggstrom-Nordin, E., Hanson, U. and Tyden, T. (2005) 'Associations between pornography consumption and sexual practices among adolescents in Sweden', *International Journal of STD and AIDS,* 16, 2, 102–107.

Haggstrom-Nordin, E. and others (2006) '"It's everywhere": young Swedish people's thoughts and reflections about pornography', *Scandanavian Journal of Caring Sciences,* 20, 4, 386–393.

Hald, G. (2006) 'Gender differences in pornography consumption among young heterosexual Danish adults', *Archive of Sexual Behavior,* 35, 5, 577–585.

Hald, G. and Malamuth, N. (2008) 'Self perceived effects of pornography consumption', *Archive of Sexual Behavior* 37, 4, 614–625.

Holland, J. and others 'Achieving masculine sexuality: young men's strategies for managing vulnerability', in Doyal, L., Naidos, J. and Wilton, T. (eds) (1994) *AIDS: setting a feminist agenda.* Taylor & Francis, London.

Kennedy, K. and Limmer, M. (2007) *Young People, Alcohol and Sexual Health: The Impact of Aspiration and Self esteem*. Rochdale: Rochdale Teenage Pregnancy Strategy.

Limmer, M. (in progress) *The Impact of Masculinity on the Sexual Decision Making of Young Men*. Lancaster: University of Lancaster.

Peter, J. and Valkenburg, P.M. (2006) 'Adolescents' exposure to sexually explicit online materials and recreational attitudes towards sex', *Journal of Communication*, 56, 4, 639–660.

Peter, J. and Valkenburg, P.M. (2007) 'Adolescents' exposure to a sexualised media environment and their notion of women as sex objects', *Sex Roles*, 56, 5–6, 381–395.

Redgrave, K. and Limmer, M. (2004) *"It Makes You More Up For It": School Aged Young People's Perspectives on Alcohol and Sexual Health*. Rochdale: Rochdale Teenage Pregnancy Strategy.

Redgrave, K. and Limmer, M. (2006) *Power, Gender and Consent: Making Sense of Sexual Risk Taking among Vulnerable Young Women*. Rochdale: Rochdale Teenage Pregnancy Strategy.

Renold, E. (2003) '"If you don't kiss me, you're dumped": boys, boyfriends and heterosexualised masculinities in the primary school', *Educational Review*, 55, 2, 179–194.

Tyden, T. and Rogala, C. (2004) 'Sexual behaviour among young men in Sweden and the impact of pornography', *International Journal of STD and AIDS*, 15, 9, 590–593.

Workshop 3: Parents – building bridges between parents and schools

Blake, S. and others (2001) 'Effects of a parent–child communications intervention on young adolescents' risk for early onset of sexual intercourse', *Family Planning Perspectives*, 33, 2, 52–61.

Health Development Agency (2001) *Teenage Pregnancy: An Update on Key Characteristics of Effective Interventions*. London: HDA. http://www.nice.org.uk/nicemedia/documents/teenpreg.pdf

Herts TP Partnership (2008) *Handy Guide for Parents and Carers in Hertfordshire*. Herts Teenage Pregnancy Partnership.

Workshop 4: Involving young people – using the 'Are You Getting It Right?' Pupil Audit Toolkit to consult young people on SRE

Martinez, A. and de Meza, L. (2008) *Are You Getting It Right? A Toolkit for Consulting Young People on Sex and Relationships Education*. London: National Children's Bureau.

New Secondary Curriculum Regional Subject Briefing: PSHE education (2008) QCA National Curriculum/PSHE Association/CfBT Education Trust. http://www.pshe-association.org.uk/new_curriculum.aspx (powerpoint presentation).

R U Thinking (2007) *Tracking Research, Wave 1 De-brief*. TNS. 20 March 2007.

SEF (2008) We Want More: *What young people want from sex and relationships education – Charter for change*. London: NCB.

Tell Us2. Ofsted, DfES and MORI 2007.

UK Youth Parliament (2007) *SRE: Are You Getting It?* London: UK Youth Parliament.

Workshop 5: Faith and Values – exploring SRE in a multi-faith society, looking at local case studies

Blake, S. and Katrak, Z. (2002) *Faith, Values and Sex and Relationships Education*. London: National Children's Bureau.

Office for Standards in Education (2008) *Waltham Forest Joint Area Review*, Sept 2008: London: Ofsted.

Workshop 6: 'Scored project' – working creatively, using football, to engage with vulnerable young people in SRE

Social Exclusion Unit (1999) *Teenage Pregnancy Report by the Social Exclusion Unit*, London: HMSO.

Heart of Birmingham Teaching Primary Care Trust (2008) *Sex and the City: Birmingham and Solihull*. Birmingham: Heart of Birmingham Teaching Primary Care Trust.

Workshop 7: What works? 17 Characteristics of effective sex education

Kirby, D. (2007) *Emerging Answers 2007: Research Findings on Programs to Reduce Teen Pregnancy and Sexually Transmitted Diseases*. Washington, DC: The National Campaign to Prevent Teen and Unplanned Pregnancy.

Reading list

ALLDRED, P. and DAVID, M. (2007)
Get Real About Sex: The Politics and Practice of Sex Education. Maidenhead: Open University Press.

ALLEN, E. and others (2007)
'Does the UK government's teenage pregnancy strategy deal with the correct risk factors? Findings from a secondary analysis of data from a randomised trial of sex education and their implications for policy', *Journal of Epidemiology and Community Health*, 61, 1 (Jan), 20–27.

ALLEN, L. (2005)
'"Say everything": exploring young people's suggestions for improving sexuality education', *Sex Education*, 5, 4 (Nov), 389–404.

ALLEN, L. (2005)
Sexual Subjects: Young People, Sexuality and Education. London: Palgrave Macmillan.

BAKER, P. and others (eds) (2007)
Teenage Pregnancy and Reproductive Health. London: Royal College of Obstetricians and Gynaecologists.

BEARINGER, L.H. and others (2007)
'Global perspectives on the sexual and reproductive health of adolescents: patterns, prevention, and potential', *Lancet*, (March) [Adolescent Health], 17–28.

BIDDULPH, M. (2007)
'Rules of engagement: boys, young men and the challenge of effective sex and relationships education', *Pastoral Care in Education*, 25, 3 (Sep), 24– 3.

BLAKE, S. (2008)
'There's a hole in the bucket: the politics, policy and practice of sex and relationships education', *Pastoral Care in Education*, 26, 1 (Mar), 33–41.

BLAKE, S. and KATRAK, Z. (2002)
Faith, Values and Sex and Relationships Education. London: National Children's Bureau. PSHE and Citizenship Spotlight Series.

BONELL, C. and others (2005)
'The effect of dislike of school on risk of teenage pregnancy: testing of hypotheses using longitudinal data from a randomised trial of sex education', *Journal of Epidemiology and Community Health*, 59, 3 (Mar), 223–230.

BONELL, C. and others (2006)
'Research report. Influence of family type and parenting behaviours on teenage sexual behaviour and conceptions'. *Journal of Epidemiology and Community Health*, 60, 6 (June), 502–506.

BOURTON, V. (2006)
'Sex education in school: young people's views', *Paediatric Nursing*, 18, 8 (Oct), 20–22.

COLEMAN, J. (2006)
Boys and Young Men: Developing Effective Sex and Relations Education in Schools. London: National Children's Bureau. Update of Forum Factsheet 11.

COLEMAN, L. and TESTA, A. (2007)
'Sexual health knowledge, attitudes and behaviours among an ethnically diverse sample of young people in the UK', *Health Education Journal*, 6, 1 (Mar), 68–81.

CORTEEN, K.M. (2006)
'Schools' fulfilment of sex and relationship education documentation: three school-based case studies', *Sex Education*, 6, 1 (Feb), 77–99.

DEPARTMENT FOR EDUCATION AND EMPLOYMENT (2000)
Sex and Relationship Education Guidance. London: DfEE. 0116/2000.

EMMERSON, L. (2008)
National Mapping of On-Site Sexual Health Services in Education Settings: Provision in Schools and Pupil Referral Units. London: National Children's Bureau.

HARVEY, R. (2008)
'Sex education at school', *British Journal of School Nursing*, 3, 2 (Mar/Apr), 62–64.

HILTON, G.L.S. (2007)
'Listening to the boys again: an exploration of what boys want to learn in sex education classes and how they want to be taught', *Sex Education*, 7, 2 (May), 161–174.

HIRST, J., FORMBY, E. and OWEN, J. (2006)
Pathways into Parenthood: Reflections from Three Generations of Teenage Mothers and Fathers. Sheffield: Sheffield Hallam University, Centre for Social Inclusion.

INDEPENDENT ADVISORY GROUP ON TEENAGE PREGNANCY (2008)
Independent Advisory Group on Teenage Pregnancy: Annual Report 2007/08.
London: Department for Children, Schools and Families.

INGHAM, R. (2005)
'"We didn't cover that at school": education against pleasure or education for
pleasure?' *Sex Education*, 5, 4 (Nov), 375–388.

KIPPAX, S. and STEPHENSON, N. (2005)
'Meaningful evaluation of SRE', *Sex Education*, 5, 4 (Nov), 359–373.

KIRBY, D. (2007)
*Emerging Answers 2007: Research Findings on Programs to Reduce Teen Pregnancy
and Sexually Transmitted Diseases.* Washington, DC: National Campaign to Prevent
Teen and Unplanned Pregnancy.

LEISHMAN, J. and MOIR, J. (eds) (2007)
Pre-teen and Teenage Pregnancy: A Twenty-First Century Reality. Keswick: M & K
Publishing.

MARTINEZ, A. (2005)
*Effective Learning Methods: Approaches to Teaching about Sex and Relationships
Within PSHE and Citizenship.* London: National Children's Bureau. 8pp. Forum
Factsheet 34. (Replaces Forum Factsheet 12, *Effective Learning Approaches*).

MARTINEZ, A. (2006)
Sex and Relationships Education: The Role of Schools. London: National Children's
Bureau. Highlight Series 229.

MARTINEZ, A. and COOPER, V. (2006)
Laying the Foundations: Sex and Relationships Education in Primary Schools. London:
National Children's Bureau. Spotlight Series.

MARTINEZ, A. and DE MEZA, L. (2008)
*Are You Getting It Right? A Toolkit for Consulting Young People on Sex and
Relationships Education.* London: National Children's Bureau.

MORFORD, R. and others (2006)
Sex and Relationships Education with Young People in Non-formal Settings. London:
National Children's Bureau. SEF Factsheet 36.

NAIK, A. (2008)
Everyday Conversations, Every Day. London: Parents Centre/Department for Children,
Schools and Families.

OFFICE FOR STANDARDS IN EDUCATION (2002)
Sex and Relationships. London: Ofsted. 44pp. HMI 433.

OFFICE FOR STANDARDS IN EDUCATION (2007)
Time for change? Personal, Social and Health Education. London: Ofsted. 24pp. HMI 070049.

PILCHER, J. (2005)
'School sex education: policy and practice in England 1870 to 2000', *Sex Education*, 5, 2 (May), 153–170.

REEVES, C. and others (2006)
'Sexual health services and education: young people's experiences and preferences', *Health Education Journal*, 65, 4 (Dec), 368–379.

SEF (2004)
Faith, Values and Sex and Relationships Education. London: SEF. Forum Factsheet.

SELWYN, N. and POWELL, E. (2007)
'Sex and relationships education in school: the views and experiences of young people', *Health Education*, 107, 2, 219–231.

SHEPHERD, W. (2007)
'Reducing teenage sexual risk-taking: painting a picture of young people's health', *Childright*, 236 (May), 28–31.

STRANGE, V. and others (2006)
'Sex and relationship education for 13–16 year olds: evidence from England', *Sex Education*, 6, 1 (Feb), 31–46.

TEENAGE PREGNANCY STRATEGY EVALUATION RESEARCH TEAM (2005)
Teenage Pregnancy Strategy Evaluation. Final Report Synthesis. London: TPSE.

UK YOUTH PARLIAMENT (2007)
SRE: Are You Getting It? London: UK Youth Parliament.

VINCENT, K. (2007)
'Teenage pregnancy and sex and relationship education: myths and (mis)conceptions', *Pastoral Care in Education*, 25, 3 (Sep), 16–23.

WALKER, J. and MILTON, J. (2006)
'Teachers' and parents' roles in the sexuality education of primary school children: a comparison of experiences in Leeds, UK and in Sydney, Australia', *Sex Education*, 6, 4 (Nov), 415–428.

WEAVER, H., SMITH, G. and KIPPAX, S. (2005)
'School-based sex education policies and indicators of sexual health among young people: a comparison of the Netherlands, France, Australia and the United States', *Sex Education*, 5, 2 (May), 171–188.

WESTWOOD, J. and MULLAN, B. (2006)
'Knowledge of secondary school pupils regarding sexual health education', *Sex Education*, 6, 2 (May), 151–162.

WESTWOOD, J. and MULLAN, B. (2007)
'Knowledge and attitudes of secondary school teachers regarding sexual health education in England', *Sex Education*, 7, 2 (May), 143–159.

All publications listed above are available for reference at NCB's library.

NCB's Library and Information Service has a comprehensive and multi-disciplinary collection of books, journals and reports on all aspects of children and young people's social care, health and education. It is the largest collection of resources about children and young people's issues in the UK.

NCB library also hosts the PSHE and Citizenship Information Service [PSHECIS].

The Library is open to visitors by appointment. NCB Members can use it for free, non-members for a fee of £10 per day.

Telephone: 020 7843 6008

Email: library@ncb.org.uk

ChildData: Four of NCBs databases – Catalogue, Organisations, Conferences and Events and Children in the News are available by subscription on the Web. For further information see http://www.ncb.org.uk/resources/detail.asp?PID=89

Websites

For a list of useful websites visit www.ncb.org.uk/sef

our charter
for good sex and relationships education

⇨ every child has the right to sex education in all areas
(gay, lesbian, straight, bisexual)
⇨ every child has the right to express their opinion
⇨ every child has the right to specific information, advice, counselling and support

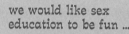

to achieve this ...

- We want Society to be more open about sex in general
- Parents should be able to talk to their children without feeling embarrassed
- There should be a special sex education team
- Teachers who feel comfortable to give sex education should be given support, courses and workshops
- Outside visitors should be allowed to come into schools

we would expect to learn about ...

- Real-life dilemmas
- Sexuality and relationship issues:
  - peer pressure
  - problems
  - friendships
  - being gay or lesbian
  - contraception
  - STIs
  - HIV
- Pros and cons about sex
  - when is the right time to have sex?
  - where to go and get advice (eg Brook)
- We would like free booklets to take away

we would like sex education to be fun ...

This would be through:
- role plays and games
- videos
- opportunities to explore dilemmas
- practising communication
- discussions that are open and multi-ethnic
- comments and suggestions box allowing pupils to ask questions who would otherwise feel embarrassed and gives us a chance to say what we want to know
- using mechanical baby dolls

we would like outside visitors to come and talk to us ...

- teenage mothers
- a lesbian or gay man
- people with different life experiences to express
- people from clinics

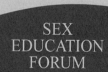

SEX
EDUCATION
FORUM

This Charter was written by young people attending a
National Children's Bureau Talkshop event on 26 February 2000.

pretty woman

love

I kissed a girl

faith

lose calories having sex

What women want

If you're not having sex you'll have no friends

sexual orientation boyfriend
shock
teen pregnancy girlfriend
puberty
everyone is
doing it

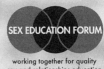

SEX EDUCATION FORUM

working together for quality
sex and relationships education

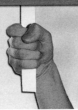

We
want
more!

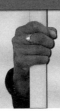

WHAT YOUNG
PEOPLE WANT
FROM SEX AND
RELATIONSHIPS
EDUCATION

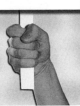

CHARTER
FOR
CHANGE

To achieve the 5 Every Child Matters outcomes, we need good sex and relationships education

To **ENJOY AND ACHIEVE** we need to learn:

- how to engage in a meaningful and fulfilling relationship.
- about the enjoyable and the positive things about sex – not just the negatives!
- what other young people have said they want to know about in SRE.
- changing feelings and emotions as we grow-up.
- about all types of relationships, allowing everyone, regardless of sexual orientation or ability, to enjoy their relationships unhindered and free from discrimination.

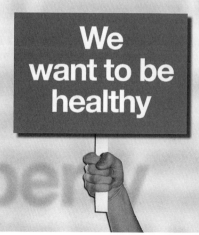

We want to be healthy

To STAY SAFE we need to learn:

- how to stand up for ourselves and be assertive in order to successfully deal with peer pressure.
- the facts about contraception and know where we can get them from, with opportunities to take part in practical demonstrations.
- the risks within the world, like the dangers of the internet, how alcohol and drugs alter our perceptions and affect our decision making.
- the types of support available for comfort and advice, and reassurance that our conversations will be treated confidentially. (If I am at risk of harm, I want to understand what will happen and who will be informed.)
- our rights and responsibilities in relationships such as the law on sex, consent and the consequences of underage sex, and how to deal with violence and rape.
- how to recognise an unsafe relationship, the signs of abuse and know if you or your friends are at risk.
- what an appropriate relationship is between family or other adults.
- other things to do to have fun and show commitment in a relationship other than having sex and how to stop things from going too far.

To **BE HEALTHY** we need to learn:

- about puberty and body changes, and the biological side of sex and reproduction.
- when we are ready for sex, and how to make decisions without being influenced or pressured by anybody or any external forces.
- about pregnancy, and all the options – termination, adoption or becoming a parent, and the emotional consequences of each choice.
- about confidential sexual health services, including in schools, clinics, GPs etc., where they are, and when they are open. Also places to go for help such as rape counselling, STI screening and LGBT support.
- about sexually transmitted infections and HIV...prevention, testing, the signs and symptoms and treatment.
- about a diverse range of relationships and how they are all natural and normal, and how to have safe sex.
- the emotional side of relationships including self confidence and self respect.

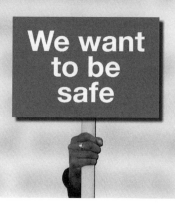

We want
to be
safe

To **ACHIEVE ECONOMIC WELL-BEING**
we need to learn:

- about pregnancy and the financial difficulties faced by young people when having a baby at an early age.
- how to get free contraception, condoms, chlamydia tests and pregnancy tests.
- how in some countries people with HIV face discrimination, and how this can affect what income they can earn.
- how young parents can get support and information about their rights, how to manage their money and avoid being poor.

To **MAKE A POSITIVE CONTRIBUTION**
we need to learn:

- how we can develop and maintain healthy relationships with everyone including our families.
- how to be able to understand other people's feelings and concerns, and help our friends if they are in trouble.
- how to help schools improve the SRE we are taught.
- how to complain if the services we use are not helpful and make suggestions to make them more young-person friendly.

OUR RECOMMENDATIONS

To make sure all children and young people receive SRE, we want schools to:

1 Make SRE (PSHE) compulsory and give it the same importance as other curriculum subjects.

2 Provide all pupils with SRE regardless of gender, ability, sexual orientation or faith and make sure the curriculum is inclusive.

3 Have better communication with young people, let them participate in setting the agenda and base SRE on their needs.

4 Make sure SRE is given a timetabled slot, is regular and that catch-up lessons are given if any are missed. SRE should be taught at appropriate stages, and start young.

5 Have better communication with parents and be more open and confident about their curriculum.

6 Let all pupils have SRE regardless of the type of school. Faith schools should not be a barrier to SRE and if they will not teach it there needs to be an alternative place to learn.

7 Make sure all staff teaching SRE are trained and have enough funding for SRE resources.

8 Teach a broad range of topics, not just about reproduction.

9 Ensure SRE is interesting, relevant and practical and is taught in a safe relaxed environment – not using scare tactics.

10 Allow teachers to give out free condoms and make sure all pupils are aware of their local sexual health clinics.

Did you know?

We asked young people between ages 16-25 to tell us about their experience of SRE in school. 1709 responded and this is what they said.

SRE is not good enough

'...one random contraceptive session in 12 months, I do not consider this to be adequate...'

Over a third of young people say said their SRE had been bad or very bad. They recognised that SRE did not have the same status as other subjects in school.

SRE is inconsistent

'Being completely unrepresented as a gay person. It was as if I didn't exist.'

Young people identifying as transgender, lesbian or gay had a worse experience of SRE, as did young people with a physical disability. The overall rating of SRE given by young people who had attended some faith schools was worse than average.

More training needed

'The teachers also were embarrassed ... they could have done with some sort of training, so they know how to tackle and explain things better.'

The quality of teaching has a huge impact on the quality of SRE experienced. Young people who said their SRE was bad also felt that their teacher did not know enough.

SRE is too biological

'I understand the science side pretty well but it seems a bit like a pencil – I know it's made from wood and soft graphite that gets broken off, but does that tell me how to write?'

Young people agree that SRE needs to include a broad range of topics. They say that whilst topics such as puberty and the biology of sex are taught, diversity of relationships, emotions relating to sex and the positive aspects of relationships are generally neglected.

SRE starts too late and is not enough

'she managed to cram all the stuff we needed to know... in year 10, which was way too late, should be in year 7 and 6.'

Young people told us that SRE had not started early enough and agreed that SRE should be introduced before the age of 13. They also said that it should not be taught as a one-off session but should be ongoing.

SRE ends too soon

'I don't see how they think that just because we're older it wouldn't be useful, considering I've only ever had one 'sex and relationships' lesson in my whole life, and that was when I was twelve.'

All young people surveyed were over 16, and around three-quarters were currently in education. Of those, four in five said that they were not currently getting any SRE. There was strong support for SRE continuing in post-16 provision, a time when most young people start becoming sexually active.

Better practice needed

'It was a rushed one-hour session with an embarrassed biology teacher. You could tell she didn't want to be there teaching us about it and didn't put us at ease at all. Everyone just took it light-heartedly and played around!'

The young people had a clear idea of what they considered good and bad practice. For example, bad SRE is taught by untrained embarrassed teachers, is not inclusive in terms of sexual orientation, and is rushed and not relevant to young people's lives. Good SRE is taught in a safe learning environment, by a non-judgemental competent educator and there is one-to-one help available after the session.

Taken from *Young people's sex and relationships education survey*. SEF 2008 (forthcoming).

Acknowledgements

This charter was written by young people participating in a Sex Education Forum residential in August 2008. It uses material written by Somerset 2BU Youth Group (LGBT) and Somerset UKYP Advisory Group. Many thanks to all the young people involved in this project.

Special thanks to UKYP for their work on this project. For more information on UKYP visit www.ukyouthparliament.org.uk

This charter was launched as part of SEF's 21st birthday celebrations.

Who is the Sex Education Forum?

The Sex Education Forum (SEF) is a collaboration of diverse organisations representing children, parents, faith, disability, health and education. We believe that all children and young people regardless of gender, faith, sexual orientation or ability are entitled to good quality sex and relationships education (SRE). SRE taught as part of a broader programme of PSHE makes a vital contribution to well-being.

Sex Education Forum
NCB
8 Wakley Street
London EC1V 7QE

Tel: 020 7843 6000
Fax: 020 7843 6053

Email: sexedforum@ncb.org.uk
Website: www.ncb.org.uk/sef

Published by the National Children's Bureau for the Sex Education Forum.

NCB
8 Wakley Street,
London EC1V 7QE

Registered Charity 258825.

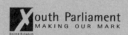